THE HUMAN EMBRYO
RESEARCH DEBATES

THE
HUMAN EMBRYO
RESEARCH DEBATES
Bioethics in the Vortex
of Controversy

RONALD M. GREEN

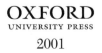

OXFORD
UNIVERSITY PRESS
2001

OXFORD
UNIVERSITY PRESS

Oxford   New York
Athens   Auckland   Bangkok   Bogotá   Buenos Aires   Calcutta
Cape Town   Chennai   Dar es Salaam   Delhi   Florence   Hong Kong   Istanbul
Karachi   Kuala Lumpur   Madrid   Melbourne   Mexico City   Mumbai
Nairobi   Paris   São Paulo   Shanghai   Singapore   Taipei   Tokyo   Toronto   Warsaw

and associated companies in
Berlin   Ibadan

Copyright © 2001 by Oxford University Press, Inc.

Published by Oxford University Press, Inc.,
198 Madison Avenue, New York, New York, 10016
http://www.oup-usa.org

Library of Congress Cataloging-in-Publication Data
Green, Ronald M.
The human embryo research debates : bioethics in the vortex of controversy /
Ronald M. Green.
p.   cm.
Includes bibliographical references and index.
ISBN 0-19-510947-3
1. Human embryo—Research—Government policy—United States.
2. Stem cells—Research—Moral and ethical aspects—United States.
I. Title.
QM608 .G74 2001   174'.25—dc21   00-053070

2 4 6 8 9 7 5 3 1

Printed in the United States of America
on acid-free paper

ACKNOWLEDGMENTS

In the course of my service as a member of the Human Embryo Research Panel I learned that the effective study of complex new issues in science and ethics requires the collaboration of people with different types of training and different points of view. This book is the result of guidance and support that I have received over the years from many such people. Of course, none of them is responsible for what I say or the positions I take.

Foremost among those to whom I owe so much are the members of the Human Embryo Research Panel. I must especially thank Steven Muller, the panel's chair, Pat King, the policy co-chair, and Brigid Hogan, the science co-chair. Working closely with Pat and Brigid, both wise leaders in their respective fields, was a great privilege. Among the panel members, my bioethics colleagues Bernie Lo, Tom Murray, and Carol Tauer, the scientist-clinician Mark Hughes, and the dedicated advocate for infertile people, Diane Aronson, have been a continuing source of education to me.

Among people at the National Institutes of Health, I would single out Sarah Carr and Duane Alexander. Sarah's energy and commitment exemplify the best in NIH staff. Duane, as head of the National Institute of Child Health & Human Development, has been a consistent advocate of better research on human reproduction.

At Dartmouth, I would like to give special thanks to Kier Olsen DeVries. Her careful reading of earlier versions of the manuscript improved my expression in many ways.

Finally, I must thank my wife Mary Jean. She was a source of support when I was a member of the Human Embryo Research Panel. Later on, while she served in the demanding post of Dean of Humanities at Dartmouth, she put up with my even longer absences in Washington as I continued my work at the NIH.

Norwich, Vermont   R. M. Green

CONTENTS

INTRODUCTION

In November 1998 a team of researchers at the University of Wisconsin led by James Thomson announced that they had been able to produce human embryonic stem (ES) cell lines. These cells have been called the "Holy Grail" of modern biology. Undifferentiated, pluripotent (capable of developing into virtually any bodily tissue), and able to proliferate indefinitely in culture, they promise to revolutionize medicine in this century. These immortalized stem cell lines may be used to replace damaged cardiac tissue following a heart attack or repair now irreversible spinal cord injuries. Parkinson's disease, Alzheimer's and diabetes are among the long list of conditions that might be cured by the ability to produce new bodily tissues.[1]

To produce the pluripotent ES cell lines, Thomson and his colleagues had to remove the inner cell mass from human embryos left over from procedures at infertility clinics. The embryos, which were stored in a frozen state, would otherwise have been thawed and discarded at some future time. Federal law forbids the National Institutes of Health (NIH) or other government agencies from funding research that involves the destruction of human embryos. As I will later explain, this ban has been in effect for more than two decades. In order to avoid violating it, Thomson had to separate his research on embryos from any public funding he received. He did this by setting up a lab in a building across campus from the facility where he does his NIH-funded research. Financial support for this duplicate laboratory came from the Geron Corporation of Menlo Park, California, which funded Thomson's work in return for an exclusive license to commercialize his discoveries.[2] Although much of the previous animal research on ES cells that had led to Thomson's achievement was federally financed, the commercial benefits would now be in private hands.

I recall reading the reports of Thomson's success with mixed feelings. In 1994, I served on the NIH's Human Embryo Research Panel, a blue ribbon group convened to recommend ethical guidelines for all future federally funded research on human embryos. The possible development of pluripotent ES cell lines was one of the reasons why the panel urged the NIH and the government to become involved in funding research on human embryos. It was therefore a pleasure to see that the promising work I had learned about almost five years before was coming to fruition. On the other hand, I was disappointed that this research had taken place under private auspices. Federal funding in this area, I knew, would not only accelerate these efforts but also prevent a handful of companies from gaining a lockhold on the basic patents likely to result.

This "privatization" of human ES cell research is only one casualty of the ban on federal support for human embryo research. The impact of this ban extends to whole areas of medical research. The field most immediately affected is reproductive medicine. In the absence of federal funding, research on the causes of infertility, miscarriages, and birth defects has been slowed. One example is research on the causes of neural tube defects. Each year thousands of children are born in this country with spina bifida and other serious neural tube malformations that lead to handicaps ranging from life-long incontinence to paraplegia. Yet it is only within the past few years that scientists have learned that a major cause of these malformations is a simple deficiency in folic acid during the earliest days of pregnancy. With this knowledge, women planning to become pregnant can now reduce the risk to their child by adding to their diet foods rich in folate or by taking inexpensive vitamin supplements.

Birth defects and stem cell research come immediately to mind as medical areas in which many people agree that more research is needed. In the wake of Thomson's announcement, the House of Representatives convened hearings to reconsider the federal ban on embryo research. Cures for Alzheimer's disease or Parkinson's disease, it seems, can stir the interest of aging congressmen.

Infertility research is another matter. A couple is considered to experience infertility when, despite their effort to have a child, they are unable to do so after a year of unprotected sex.[3] Infertility is designated as "primary" when a couple is never able to have a child and "secondary" when it is experienced after the birth of one or more children. The 1995 National Survey of Family Growth lists as "infertile" 2.1 million married women of childbearing age. This amounts to 7.1 percent of the twenty-nine million married women of childbearing age.[4] In addition to the many women who suffer from infertility, an equally large number suffers from "impaired fecundity." Although they can conceive, they are unable to carry a pregnancy to term.[5] Over all, it is estimated that as many as 10 percent of all couples experience difficulty in having children.[6]

Many of these couples experience acute distress as a result of their problems.[7] The persistent inability to have a child is frequently likened to the experience of grieving over the loss of a loved one, in this case the longed-for child.[8] Nevertheless, the problem of infertility is often downplayed or ignored. Friends and relatives blandly assure women that if they relax they will get pregnant. Few states require that infertility treatments be covered by employer insurance, while less than 20 percent of all health insurers cover *in vitro* fertilization (IVF).[9] Some bioethicists have even tried to argue that infertility is an elective use of medical care, like liposuction or breast enhancement. They maintain this even though infertility, as a major source of suffering caused by a biological abnormality, meets every criterion for being a serious illness or disease.[10] It is one reflection of the widespread indifference to this problem that despite the fact that several million Americans suffer from fertility-related problems, the NIH, the principal federal health research agency, spends less than one-tenth of 1 percent of its nearly $16 billion annual budget on infertility research.[11]

In a later chapter, I will review some of the factors that lead us to downplay the medical problem of infertility. But the federal ban on human embryo research is one immediate cause of this neglect. The ban has been in effect since the late 1970s, when the development of IVF initiated the era of modern reproductive medicine and first made possible research to study the embryo *ex utero*—outside the mother's womb. Since that time, research has gone on in privately funded infertility clinics, but it has usually been directed at improving the chances of a pregnancy. There has been far less basic research aimed at trying to understand the complex processes of conception, implantation, and embryo development—or the many ways these processes can go wrong. This kind of basic research needs government support because it is costly and because it does not usually immediately lead to the higher success rates valued by privately funded clinics. Since the late 1970s federal support has been blocked by a combination of outright bans, deliberate neglect, and tentative but ultimately unsuccessful efforts at change.

The Human Embryo Research Panel is one of those failed efforts. During the year I served on the panel, I learned that basic research in reproductive medicine can make enormous contributions to alleviating infertility. It can also improve understanding and treatment of many other disease conditions, including childhood cancers and birth defects. Embryo research is a precondition to valuable work on stem cells and embryonic gene therapy. For all these reasons, the panel strongly recommended federal support for this research area. Nevertheless, the panel's recommendations went largely unheeded. By the end of 1994, the White House began to back away from our work. In the following year, a resurgent conservative Congress began the process of reimposing a formal ban on embryo research that remains in effect today.

Although I feel enormously privileged to have worked with so many outstanding scientists, physicians, and policy experts during that year, I emerged from the experience with a sense of despair. Opposition by anti-abortion activists along with widespread public ignorance or indifference to the issues have caused one of the most basic and promising areas of biomedical research to be excluded from federal support. The privatization of James Thomson's stem cell research is one consequence of this exclusion. Another is the fact that in the area of reproductive medicine, the United States is becoming a "debtor" nation, dependent for progress on research performed in countries like Great Britain, where there is a more supportive legal environment.

The most immediate and tragic consequence of this lack of federal support is the epidemic of serious birth complications caused by poorly researched but widely used infertility procedures. In the absence of federal funding, reproductive medicine has not come to a halt. Problems of infertility, some created by the tendency to marry later in life and the development of new treatments, have stimulated the growth of this industry such that, as of January 1999, 356 infertility clinics were in operation throughout the United States.[12] Without the kinds of basic research needed to establish the safety and efficacy of new procedures, women, children, and families are often placed at risk.

A leading problem is the virtual epidemic of multiple births—twins, triplets, and more.[13] This results from the use of powerful drugs to stimulate a woman to develop a number of fertilizable eggs and from the practice of transferring numerous embryos to the uterus in order to improve a woman's chances of becoming pregnant. According to statistics gathered in a 1995 study by the Centers for Disease Control and Prevention, 37 percent of pregnancies resulting from IVF and related assisted reproductive technologies resulted in a multiple birth, compared with 2 percent of the general population.[14] Beyond the media coverage of happy parents of sextuplets and octuplets, these practices have greatly increased the number of very sick premature infants in neonatal intensive care units around the country. Clinicians are not solely to blame for this problem. Couples who pay for these procedures often willingly invite the risks rather than fail in their efforts to start a family. A generation of children with birth-related cerebral palsy, mental retardation, and severe respiratory or digestive problems is a little-noted consequence of the practice of infertility medicine *and* the ban on human embryo research.

To some extent, reproductive medicine and human embryo research are casualties of our cultural wars. Opposition to abortion is one factor that has slowed progress in these areas. Many who hold the view that life is sacred from conception onward feel compelled to resist research and clinical practices that require the routine manipulation or destruction of human embryos. But the problem goes deeper than this. New scientific and technical developments are raising questions that push the boundaries of our accustomed modes of ethical thinking. The difficulty of answering these questions leads some to resist doing so. They prefer to content themselves with older, easier answers, even when those answers no longer fit the choices we face and have the effect of impeding progress and research. Others are willing to address the questions but, confused by their novelty and complexity, end by ceding to those who loudly defend the older positions.

Many examples of these kinds of troubling questions exist. One is, "When does human life begin?" Many people who oppose abortion quickly reply, "At the moment of conception." But in response to this familiar answer, biological research raises a new question: "What do you mean by 'the moment of conception?'" Research shows that conception (fertilization) involves a "complex sequence of coordinated events" stretching over hours or even days.[15] At what point in this sequence can we say that something morally or spiritually decisive has happened? How we can find bright moral lines when nature offers only continuous biological processes? Our increasing ability to study every step in the early development of the embryo sharpens these question. Those unwilling to be challenged by them retreat to more comforting answers from the past. No longer an answer to a question, the statement "Life begins at conception" becomes a refusal to consider the question at all.

Another example of the way in which biological research and knowledge are pushing the boundaries of our accustomed modes of ethical thinking consists of the issue of "potentiality." It is common for opponents of human embryo research to base their valuation of the embryo on its "potentiality" for development into a full human being. However, both stem cell and cloning research have radically recast the issues. With some degree of technical intervention, virtually any cell in the human body now has the "potential" to become a child. Does this mean that every cell merits full protection and may not be used in research? If it is objected that a stem or body cell's potentiality to become a human being is highly artificial and depends on intensive technological intervention, the same might be said of the embryos created in IVF procedures. They, too, will never realize their "potentiality" without highly artificial technological manipulations. The deeper question here is how we are even to think about something like "potentiality" in such a rapidly changing scientific environment.

Our increasing powers of control over reproduction and human biological development raise other difficult new ethical and philosophical questions. The advent of IVF helps women with blocked oviducts to have children. With the help of intracytoplasmic sperm injection (ICSI, pronounced "ICK-see"), men who produce no viable sperm can now become fathers. Couples who previously avoided reproduction because they feared transmitting serious inherited genetic disorders to their offspring can now use preimplantation genetic diagnosis (PGD or PID) to select for healthy embryos even before pregnancy begins. Promising new technologies such as embryonic gene therapy are in prospect. Somatic cell nuclear transfer (cloning) lies on the horizon as a reproductive alternative for some individuals or couples who produce no sex cells at all.

But none of these technologies is risk-free. Some evidence exists, for example, that ICSI may lead to a higher rate of chromosomal abnormalities in the resulting children.[16] One recent study suggests that DNA from viruses carried into the egg by this invasive technology may cause heritable genetic mutations in the resulting children.[17] Already mentioned are the possible risks of IVF. Even when undertaken by the best of laboratories, preimplantation genetic diagnosis can result in errors and the birth of children with severe genetic disorders. Cloning risks the birth of a child whose cells have already aged and whose life span may be shortened.[18] All these technologies raise the unfamiliar question of how much risk we are justified in imposing on our children as the price of having them. Is it ever permissible to risk a child's physical health and quality of life in order to bring it into being? If we conclude that it is not ethical to do so and demand the most stringent standards of protection for children born as a result of reproductive procedures—a standard of "no risk to the future child"—we threaten to close down progress in this entire area of medicine. However, if we hold that parents have a right to try to have children despite the risks, we may help produce a generation of damaged people. In research contexts, the challenge is to identify an appropriate level of risk when the very existence of the research subject depends on our decisions. Does such research amount to "unethical experiments on the unborn," as some have argued, or does it represent a reasonable accommodation to risk in view of the benefits to parents, society, and perhaps the children themselves?

My aim in this book is to introduce some of the most important implications of the new reproductive and genetic possibilities and explore the perplexing ethical questions they raise. I also want to shed light on the array of social forces, conceptual problems, and organized opposition groups that have worked together to stall human embryo research. To do this, I have chosen to retrace the steps in my own learning process by beginning with an extended account of my year of service on the Human Embryo Research Panel. During that year, the panel was introduced to some of the surprising new information being generated by researchers in human embryology and genetics. Among other things, we learned that a broad new field of biomedicine is emerging that involves a union of reproductive medicine with genetic science. One writer has termed this field "reprogenetics."[19] Against this background, the members of the Human Embryo Research Panel had to develop new ways of thinking about the ethical questions these possibilities raise. With the NIH's request for guidance always before us, we had to fit our answers into a framework that made sense for public policy. Finally, we had to do this in the vortex of Washington's press and politics.

The account of the panel's work with which I begin is more than a chronological narrative of the year's events. It is better described as a "philosophical memoir." Interspersed with descriptions of Beltway politics and cultural strife that constantly impinged on our work are extended theoretical reflections in which I try to review my thinking on some of the leading ethical issues underlying the surface controversies.

The work of the Human Embryo Research Panel was not an isolated event. It was preceded by almost two decades of ethical reviews of embryo research and the work of other panels, both in the United States and abroad, that have tried to forge policies to govern this area. In the few years since the panel issued its report, embryo research has once again drawn public attention in connection with newly developed cloning and stem cell technologies. Thus, the "embryo research debates" go on. In the final chapters of this book I try to bring these issues up to date. Drawing on some of my continuing Washington service in relation to these issues, I show how the same basic ethical, political, and religious problems revealed in the work of the panel continue to shape our national controversies.

I hope that by taking the reader along with me on this journey into public reproductive bioethics, I can convey its importance and confer an understanding of the forces working both to accelerate and impede progress. I personally believe that federally funded, ethically regulated research on human embryos is a central component of modern biomedicine. As Thomson's stem cell work shows, embryo research is the gateway to expanding our knowledge of the most basic cellular and genetic processes in human beings. Despite this, embryo research remains the sole major area of biomedical investigation that has been repeatedly blocked by political interference and that remains off-limits for federal support. The time has come to bring this extended period of research obstruction to an end.

THE HUMAN EMBRYO
RESEARCH DEBATES

1

INTO THE VORTEX

THE story of my encounter with the science and ethics of human embryo research begins in early January 1994. Dartmouth's winter term classes had just begun. Julie Wright, my administrative assistant at the Ethics Institute, told me that I had received a call from the office responsible for science policy and technology transfer at the National Institutes of Health (NIH). "It's about serving on a panel they're forming dealing with embryos, fetuses, or something," said Julie.

Returning the call, I remember trying to think my way through Julie's imprecision. "Maybe this is about fetal tissue research," I speculated. The year before, in one of the first acts of his administration, President Clinton had used his executive power to authorize the use of tissues from aborted fetuses as a source of transplant material for research on Parkinson's disease, diabetes, and other disorders. That policy had been recommended five years earlier by a special NIH panel, but the Bush administration had not implemented it.[20] Nevertheless, the connection to fetal tissue research made no sense. "That matter has been resolved," I told myself. "Why is the NIH forming a new panel?"

Sarah Carr, a young administrator at the Office of Science Policy, began to answer my questions. With the arrival of preparatory materials over the next few weeks, I realized that, along with eighteen other members of the Human

1

Embryo Research Panel, I was about to embark on a challenging journey. Our subject was not fetuses, but human embryos: the tiny multicellular organisms resulting from the fertilization of egg by sperm. As a result of Clinton's action the year before, the NIH and federal government already had regulations in place governing research on fetuses, which are defined as the "product of conception from the time of implantation (as evidenced by the presumptive signs of pregnancy)."[21] What were lacking entirely were regulations governing research on *ex utero* embryos (those outside and not yet implanted in a womb) that are being produced by the thousands in infertility clinics around the world by means of in vitro fertilization (IVF).

The preparatory materials sent to me helped fill in the historical blanks. More than fifteen years before, on 25 July, 1978, modern infertility medicine began with the birth in Oldham and General District Hospital in the north of England of Louise Brown, the world's first "test tube" baby. For the first time in history, human embryos could be created outside the womb, studied during their earliest phases of growth, and then returned to the womb for gestation and birth. The development of IVF not only made the early, *ex utero* embryo a possible research "subject," but the rapid growth of infertility medicine created demand for better, more successful infertility treatments. Since 1978 a variety of new assisted reproductive technologies (ARTs) have developed. Most involve intensive clinical efforts and considerable expense, little of it covered by health insurance. In the United States alone, over 60,000 IVF procedures are being performed every year.[22] Popular magazines and books are filled with stories about the enormous frustration experienced by couples trying to start a family using technologies like IVF or intracytoplasmic sperm injection (ICSI).[23] In some cases, homes have been mortgaged to pay the tens of thousands of dollars these procedures cost the couples.[24] Women undergo painful and emotionally stressful drug treatments. Despite this, more often than not, no birth results.

Reading the preparatory material, I learned that in the late 1970s, following the first successes with IVF in England and the United States, Congress created an Ethics Advisory Board (EAB) to recommend and apply guidelines for federally funded research in this area. In May 1979, after months of study, discussions, and public hearings, the EAB issued a report recommending support for a gamut of research using human embryos.[25] This included permission for the deliberate creation of embryos for research purposes only, even when there was no intention of transferring the resulting embryos to a womb. The EAB's deliberations and its report stirred enormous controversy. The opportunity for public comment following release of the report produced nearly 13,000 letters, all but three hundred of them opposed to *in vitro* fertilization research. Many of these letters reflected organized protest campaigns undertaken by religious groups.[26]

As it turns out, no action was ever taken on the report. Joseph A. Califano, Jr., then secretary of health, education and welfare (HEW), published the EAB report for public discussion, but in September 1979 he resigned from his position. No subsequent secretary of HEW or Health and Human Services (HHS) took up the issue.[27] When the board's charter expired in 1979, its membership was not renewed and no funding was provided. Since U.S. law required that all research in this area supported by the NIH or other federal agencies be reviewed by the EAB, the result was a *de facto* moratorium on federal support for embryo research in this country. During the Reagan and Bush years, despite efforts to end it by various NIH and HHS administrators,[28] this moratorium was maintained because both administrations were aligned with "right-to-life" constituencies that opposed any manipulations of human embryos. Research on embryos and infertility procedures continued in privately funded infertility clinics around the country, but it was often limited by the immediate need to produce pregnancies. For fifteen years, progress in infertility medicine and embryo research in this country was slowed by America's abortion politics.

During this period, some basic research went forward overseas. In the mid-1980s, a British commission chaired by Dame Mary Warnock recommended government funding for IVF and embryo research. The result was a voluntary licensing authority that oversaw infertility clinics and IVF research projects in the United Kingdom. In 1990, after several years of building trust with clinicians, researchers, and the public through the voluntary program, the Human Fertilisation and Embryology Authority (HFEA), an official government agency, was brought into being to provide oversight and guidance for clinical and research programs in infertility medicine. During this period Australia, too, had significant IVF and embryo research programs, although more recently its state legislatures, responding to pressure from religious groups, began to pass laws restricting the use of embryos in research.

My hunch proved right that a changed attitude toward reproductive medicine, ushered in by the Clinton administration, was behind the formation of the Human Embryo Research Panel. In June 1993, encouraged by the fetal tissue initiative and prodded by supporters of infertility research at the NIH's Institute of Child Health & Human Development, Congress passed a law, a provision of the NIH Revitalization Act, that nullified the requirement of EAB approval of federal funding for infertility and embryo research projects.[29] For the first time in fifteen years, the NIH was free to respond to research proposals in this area. More than forty of these proposals were already in the pipeline. However, before approving any of them, senior NIH administrators felt they needed guidelines to instruct members of Institutional Review Boards (IRBs), the local bodies at universities and research institutions charged with approving human subject and fetal tissue research. In late 1993 these developments led to a decision by senior NIH administrators to form the Human Embryo Research Panel. This was the group on which I was now being asked to serve.

The first meeting of the panel took place several weeks later, on 2 and 3 February 1994, in a large function room at the Pooks Hill Marriott Hotel in Bethesda, Maryland. Over the years, I had served on many NIH peer-review study sections for grant proposals having to do with genetic research. These also met in one or another Bethesda hotel, but this first meeting of the embryo panel was different. The crowd of press, NIH and other federal officials, and observers from the general public was the first sign to me that, despite the passage of fifteen years since the work of the EAB, human embryo research was as controversial as ever. As I entered the large conference room where we were meeting, it struck me for the first time that this was no routine ethics review panel, but a group placed at the center of one of society's most divisive and controversial debates. I was to learn that along with the privileged position of being a panel member (which included the right to sit at the center table and to ask questions or speak whenever one wished), there were to be some legal and possibly even physical risks.

The panel had nineteen members from a variety of backgrounds. Three of the members (John Eppig, Andrew Hendrickx, and Brigid Hogan, our science co-chair) were doing research in mammalian embryology. Six were physicians. Of these, four (Patricia Donahoe, Mary Martin, Kenneth Ryan, and Mark Hughes) worked in the area of reproductive medicine, one (Fernando Guerra) had a primary interest in public health, and the sixth, Bernard Lo, focused on medical ethics. Three of the other members (Tom Murray, Carol Tauer, and myself) were biomedical ethicists. Two (Alta Charo and panel policy co-chair Pat King) were lawyers. One member (Dorothy Nelkin) was a sociologist, and two (panel chair Stephen Muller, former president of The Johns Hopkins University, and Nan Keohane, president of Duke University) were political scientists. Rounding out the group were two other members (Diane Aronson and Ola Huntley) who belonged to constituencies with an interest in the panel's work. Diane was head of Resolve, an organization dedicated to helping couples with infertility. Ola, of African American background, was the mother of a child with sickle cell anemia, a severe genetic disease that might be treated by preimplantation genetic diagnosis or embryonic gene therapy, both of which required embryo research.

Apart from the diversity and depth of our expertise, there was no obvious reason why any of us had been chosen for this task. I suspect my institutional position and prior service in grant review panels for the genome program may have played a role, but this is speculation. It might have been my background in religious ethics that was of interest to the NIH. Later, as our work got under way, the panel's composition became a major source of controversy.

Critics complained of the lack of "pro-life" representation and were not appeased by the fact that two of the three academic bioethicists (Tom Murray and Carol Tauer) were of Roman Catholic background. Carol, a former nun, was teaching at the College of St. Catherine, a Roman Catholic institution. Repeated charges were made that the panel was stacked with researchers and clinicians seeking funding for their work on human embryos. In fact, only three of the panel members (Mark Hughes, Mary Martin, and Patricia Donahoe) were actually working in areas that might receive support if federal funding of human embryo research were approved. Their presence was consistent with the NIH peer-review system. This system relies on experts in each scientific field to evaluate research proposals and approve research directions. Efforts are made to avoid immediate conflicts of interest. For example, a scientist is not allowed to review a collaborator's grant proposal. Nevertheless, the requirement that peer reviewers have expertise in the field often gives them a stake in its direction and in federal support for it.

Could the NIH have done more to balance the panel and protect it from these charges? Possibly. The Human Fetal Tissue Transplantation Research Panel in 1988 included at least several publicly recognized representatives of a "pro-life" position. This representation moderated the force of the charge that the panel had been stacked. But it hardly assuaged the most vehement critics, who rejected the panel's majority recommendations, and it resulted in several sharp dissents from the panel's recommendations—including one that was longer than the panel report itself.[30] Lack of consensus here probably weakened the panel's ultimate recommendations.[31]

Did NIH administrators, therefore, deliberately try to create an embryo research panel that would approve research without dissent? I see nothing to support this charge. Apart from the diversity and depth of our expertise, there was no obvious reason why any of us had been chosen. In a letter written in reply to congressional inquiries, Sandy Chamblee, acting deputy director of the Office of Science Policy and Technology Transfer, stated that panel members were selected not "as proponents of specific viewpoints" but "for their knowledge, expertise, experience, perspectives, and for the thoughtful and careful approach they would take in fulfilling their important and sensitive assignment."[32] She emphasized that no members had been polled in advance for their views about the acceptability of embryo research. As far as I know, these are accurate statements. Before the telephone call from Sarah Carr, no one at the NIH had spoken to me about the panel. No NIH administrator or staff person ever revealed any knowledge of my prior writings in reproductive ethics. The same is true for Carol Tauer. Although in her published work Carol had been moving toward some newer Catholic views that attribute lesser moral status to very early embryo, she had no fixed or established position on this or the topic of embryo research. She seems to have been chosen primarily because she was a respected Roman Catholic ethicist and a woman. Reflecting on her own appointment and that of other panel members in a later essay, Carol supported my own perception of how the NIH proceeded when she observed that "at the time of appointment none of us was asked whether we did or did not support IVF or human embryo research."[33]

That first meeting day, February 2, proved enormously important in shaping the direction our work would take. The day opened with remarks by Harold Varmus, the Nobel Prize-winning physician and scientist who had been appointed director of the NIH only a few months before. After briefly reviewing the history leading to the panel's formation, Varmus told us that our task was to consider and provide advice to the federally chartered advisory committee to the director (ACD) about various areas of research involving the human embryo. The ACD would, in turn, make a recommendation to him that could form the basis for further administrative regulations governing NIH practice. Following a period for public comment, these recommendations would go into effect. Varmus told us that we were to divide our recommendations into three categories: research areas that we judged to be acceptable for federal funding, those that warranted additional review, and those that were unacceptable. Varmus offered no explanation of these categories. He indicated that he would like to have our recommendations in place for the June meeting of the ACD. He also told us that we were not to consider the issue of germ-line gene therapy. This research area, which involves the insertion of corrected gene sequences into embryos that would otherwise be affected by serious genetic disorders, would be considered at some future time by a separate body more suited to review the special issues of genetic research. Months down the line, as we finally organized our recommendations, we would devote considerable time to deciding what "additional review" meant and what forms it might take. As it turns out, we would not see Varmus himself again until December, when our work was completed. At that time, events would reveal the depth of his commitment not only to the panel process he helped initiate but to scientific freedom, as well.

The principal speaker at our first meeting was Jonathan Van Blerkom, a reproductive endocrinologist with clinical and research experience in infertility medicine. Van Blerkom's presentation introduced us to the subject of our panel's work, the "preimplantation embryo." This is the tiny entity that exists in the two-week period following the events of conception. Though normally hidden in darkness as it travels down a woman's fallopian tube to the uterus, it is now routinely subject to examination and research in infertility programs, where conception and the first days of its development occur entirely outside the body. In one sense, the term "preimplantation embryo" is a misnomer. Implantation normally occurs at about six to seven days of development *in vivo*. Since we would eventually permit research on *in vitro* embryos up to fourteen days old, some of these would be "postimplantation" embryos in a strictly chronological sense. However, existing federal regulations to protect the fetus define it as "the product of conception from the time of implantation."[34] These regulations are directed at research on fetuses in their mother's womb or after they are aborted. They do not cover *in vitro* embryos, which, in this legal sense, are "preimplantation embryos." Some researchers preferred to call this entity the "pre-embryo"[35] to distinguish it from the significantly changed being that makes its appearance with the development of the primitive streak at about two weeks gestational age. However, this term has been subject to criticism by anti-abortion groups as diminishing the early embryo's moral claims. To avoid this controversy, we chose the technically imperfect but more neutral term *preimplantation embryos*.

The day's briefing materials gave us enough of an overview of embryo development to help us understand Van Blerkom's and others' science presentations. (See Appendix A for a schematic summary of human embryogenesis). We learned that following fertilization, the embryo takes the form of a single-cell zygote. Repeated cell divisions over the next few days lead to a compact collection of early cells known as "blastomeres." At this stage the embryo is sometimes called the "morula," a Latin term that literally means "mulberry." At about four to six days development, with the embryo about a tenth of a millimeter in size (about the size of the period at the end of this sentence), an outer layer of these cells begins to differentiate into the "trophoblast" cell type that eventually becomes placental material needed to sustain the embryo's growth. The remaining cells, called the "inner cell mass" (ICM) cluster at the center of the embryo. A fluid-filled void appears at the center of the embryo, now termed a "blastocyst." Up to this point, the embryo has been traveling down one of the fallopian tubes toward the uterus. At about six days of development, the blastocyst reaches the womb and implantation begins. Cell division continues, but the next distinctive events occur at about two weeks of gestational age. At that time, the implanted embryo still consists of a disk of undifferentiated cells, surrounded by trophoblasts, or early placental material. Within this embryonic disk, a small cluster of cells forms an organizing center that soon becomes a line down the disk's middle, the so-called "primitive streak." This marks the beginning of a process known as "gastrulation." Under the microscope, the primitive streak appears as an indentation that evidences massive cellular movements. It quickly gives rise to three layers of specialized cells that eventually form all the tissues and organs of the body. From this point forward, the embryo begins constructing the specialized tissues and organs that form a human being. This process of "organogenesis" continues until eight weeks of gestational age, when most of the major organ systems will have made their appearance. At this stage, the developing embryo technically becomes a "fetus."

Van Blerkom's presentation opened before us an area of research that simultaneously displayed great feats of scientific ingenuity and surprising gaps in knowledge. He began by signaling the pressing need to go beyond animal research in this area. Over the years, he told us, scientists had developed a large body of detailed knowledge about embryo development in frogs, mice, cows, and rabbits. Much of this research suggested clinical directions in infertility medicine and elsewhere that might apply to human beings. But there was a problem: in many ways the human embryo is different from other species, and its path of development is unique. This is true even among primates. For example, we later learned that even though early rubella vaccination research in monkeys indicated that the vaccine did not cross the placenta, subsequent research in humans showed otherwise. Since exposure to the rubella virus can seriously damage a developing fetus, this made the vaccine unsafe for human use.[36]

The core of Van Blerkom's presentation was a series of slides of eggs and embryos produced in his and others' infertility laboratories. We learned that clinicians around the world had struggled for years with the problem of grading eggs and embryos for use in infertility procedures. Since women being treated frequently produce more eggs than are needed, and many of these eggs, when fertilized, will produce embryos, the urgent question before clinicians is, "Which embryos should we return to the womb?" Not all embryos have the same degree of "developmental competence." Some will cleave, dividing into two, four, or eight cells, and so on, and continue to develop normally, while others will simply stop dividing after several cell divisions. Some will continue to develop, but because of very serious physical, chromosomal, or genetic abnormalities may lead to later abortion or the birth of a child with serious abnormalities. One example is the phenomenon of polyploidy, in which two (or more) sperm penetrate the egg. A resulting "triploid" embryo has three, rather than the normal two, sets of chromosomes. This condition is incompatible with life, and the embryo/fetus usually dies before birth. In lesser forms, in which only a single chromosome pair is affected, such as in trisomy 21 (Down syndrome), excess chromosomes can lead to severe retardation and other birth defects.

This grading problem is a serious one. Obviously, no one knowingly wants to start a pregnancy that will lead to stillbirth or a child with birth defects, nor do clinicians want to return too many embryos to the womb, since this can lead to twin, triplet, or even higher-order multiple births with serious health risks for the resulting children.[37] So the question "Which are the best eggs to fertilize and the best embryos to transfer?" is of more than academic interest. What Van Blerkom's presentation showed is that despite more than fifteen years of practice of IVF by hundreds of clinics around the world, nobody has a very clear idea of what makes eggs or embryos good or bad. Most grading systems rely on microscopic observation of the cells' structures and form. But these systems often have little relation to developmental competence. Many perfectly "normal looking" embryos inexplicably stop dividing after one or two cell divisions. In contrast, some embryos with gross abnormalities in the cytoplasm, including darkened regions or voids, go on to produce perfectly normal children.[38] Research had even shown that some polyspermic and triploid embryos could produce normal children. Was this the result of unknown corrective mechanisms by which the extra chromosomes are ejected as the embryo develops? No one knew.

Van Blerkom emphasized that this poor understanding of egg and embryo competence has several serious implications for reproductive medicine. First, it meant that in clinics around the world, many eggs and embryos that could be used to produce healthy, normal children were routinely being discarded on the basis of poorly researched grading criteria. This meant that some women were being subjected to more cycles of powerful infertility medications than were needed. Others were being deprived of the opportunity to use eggs or embryos that might produce children. All this contributed to the cost and inefficiency of these procedures.

Why, after almost fifteen years of clinical practice, was reproductive medicine so little advanced in a matter that one would think was basic to good clinical practice? Van Blerkom's answer was blunt: much of the research in this field was "awful." Rather than being undertaken by laboratory-based investigators with a good understanding of other mammalian studies, research was often "empirical." In the effort to improve immediate pregnancy outcomes, clinicians or laboratory personnel tried to manipulate different parameters of a treatment program, such as the growth media used to culture embryos. But, in the absence of government support, there was not enough money available for systematic collaboration among different clinics, and the small numbers of embryos used in existing research protocols often rendered results invalid. Looking back at nearly 700 published studies since the advent of IVF, Van Blerkom offered a very negative judgment. Because they were "poorly designed" and lacked adequate controls, he said, many of these studies "basically conflict with one another."

The problem was not just the inefficiency of infertility procedures. Experimental treatments also created unknown but possibly significant risks for the children produced by them. Van Blerkom offered an illustration from one of the more promising infertility procedures being developed, one known as "assisted hatching." Human beings, no less than birds or reptiles, hatch out of eggs. This takes place in the first days of embryonic development, when the growing embryo, preparing to implant in the lining of the womb, bursts out of the zona pellucida that, until that point, has kept the individual cells together. On the theory that some embryos fail to develop because their zona is too tough, clinicians had begun using microsurgical techniques to pierce the membrane of some eggs before returning them to the uterus. Van Blerkom noted that recent studies of embryos that failed to hatch had found a very high incidence of chromosomal and other abnormalities in these embryos. Could it be that hatching is one of the obstacles that nature imposes to test the developmental competence of embryos? Might the assisted hatching procedure, by circumventing this natural checkpoint, lead to a higher incidence of birth defects? In the absence of systematic, multicenter studies of these questions, no one knew. Meanwhile, in reproductive clinics around the world, well-meaning clinicians continued their piecemeal, and possibly harmful, efforts to help infertile couples.

More recently, a similar problem has been reported with an even more advanced technology now widely in use, intracytoplasmic sperm injection (ICSI). In many respects, this is a "miracle cure" for many infertile couples. Research indicates that up to 30 percent of infertility is caused by male-factor problems. Another 30 percent is traceable to female problems, and 40 percent is unexplained.[39] In the past, couples in which the male had a low sperm count or did not produce viable sperm could resort only to sperm donation or adoption to have a family. With ICSI, however, clinicians can take a single sperm and, using micromanipulation techniques, inject it directly into the woman's egg. When the husband is unable to ejaculate motile sperm, immature sperm cells can be taken from the sperm-producing layer (epididymis) of the testis. Thanks to ICSI, thousands of couples around the world who were infertile have now been able to have their own biological children. The fact remains, however, that ICSI is a highly invasive procedure. In normal fertilization, only genetic material from the head of the sperm penetrates the egg, but when ICSI is used, the entire sperm is physically inserted. No one is entirely sure that this process does not disrupt the delicate structural or genetic material of the egg.[40] A recent study on monkeys has shown that foreign DNA can be inserted into embryos using ICSI.[41] Will the same thing happen as a result of the clinical practice of ICSI, with sperm-borne viruses entering into human DNA and resulting in a host of new inherited genetic diseases in human populations? A further problem is that because genetic or chromosomal problems sometimes contribute to male infertility, sperm from infertile men may have a higher incidence of genetic problems that could be passed on to the resulting embryo and child. Another recent study indicates that there is a slight but significant increase in the rate of spontaneous sex-chromosome anomalies among children born as a result of ICSI compared with the general newborn population.[42] These possibilities have led some observers to urge early prenatal genetic testing for all women who have conceived babies through ICSI.[43]

All these problems identified by Van Blerkom lead to an obvious question: Is infertility medicine worth the current "costs"? Should we permit the use of poorly studied treatments? Maybe the solution to these problems is not to increase support for better research but to impose stricter limits on infertility medicine itself. One does not have to speculate about the effects of experimental technologies like assisted hatching or ICSI to arrive at this conclusion. A good deal of evidence exists that many common assisted reproductive procedures are harmful to children. I already mentioned one of the most pressing and serious problems; the epidemic of multiple births—twins, triplets, and more—now evident in Europe and the United States.[44] In an effort to produce pregnancies, physicians and clinics administer high doses of stimulatory medication and sometimes return three or more embryos to women's wombs. This has resulted in a documented thirty to thirty-fivefold increase in the number of dizygotic (fraternal) twin deliveries and a corresponding increase in even higher-order multiple births.[45] This epidemic of multiple births has become one of the leading iatrogenic—physician-caused—health problems in the industrialized world. Some efforts have been made to reduce the risk. British regulations limit to three the number of embryos that may be transferred, and some U. S. bodies that have studied the issue have urged similar limits.[46] Nevertheless, patients or couples frequently place the opportunity for a pregnancy ahead of the risk and tend to resist such limits.[47]

Problems like these are fodder for many critics of the assisted reproductive technologies. A diverse assortment of people with very different points of view on reproductive matters is united in opposition to these technologies. During the early 1990s I worked with a colleague from Dartmouth's infertility clinic and another from the psychology department to offer a multidisciplinary undergraduate course on the "ethical, legal, and social challenges of assisted reproduction." We found that much of the content of the course was devoted to examining these objections. At one end of the spectrum of critical opinion is the Roman Catholic church. Despite its generally pro-natalist position, official Catholic teaching is opposed to almost all assisted reproductive procedures.[48] This is because of its view of the sanctity of the early human embryo and its position that every child has a "right" to be born through a natural act of sexual intercourse between its (married) parents. At the opposite end of the spectrum are some feminists who see the new assisted reproductive technologies as an extension of male-dominated medicine and an effort to technologize and control women's reproduction.[49] One leading feminist critic, sociologist Barbara Katz Rothman, regards the effort to have a biologically related child as an expression of outmoded patriarchal views about the importance of male lineage and the "male seed."[50] Between these positions we find people who have no particular view of infertility but who fear the possible eugenic manipulations to which new reproductive technologies might lead. Others see infertility medicine as a costly luxury available only to privileged white couples in countries where many members of minority groups lack basic health care.[51] Some critics ask why costly infertility medicine is needed in a world of overpopulation and environmental crisis.[52]

Preparing for that course led me to disagree with many of the critics of reproductive medicine. Infertility, I came to believe, is a genuine disease condition. Although not life threatening, it fits the best definition of disease: a failure of function of a major bodily system that causes death, disability or suffering.[53] Admittedly, no one dies from being infertile, but it is often a great source of emotional suffering. Infertile women have been found to be more depressed than fertile women, with levels of psychological distress as high as women with cancer and heart disease.[54] In one group of interviews with couples undergoing IVF, half the women described infertility as the most upsetting experience of their lives.[55] If we consider that other non-life-threatening physical problems that cause emotional distress, from acne to cleft lip, are deserving of medical treatment, it is hard to see why infertility treatments should be singled out for criticism. The point that infertility is a medical problem hardly needs to be made any longer in the wake of the enthusiastic reception given Viagra by patients and physicians.[56] Although erectile dysfunction (ED) certainly merits medical treatment, no one can say that infertility is a less serious medical problem.

Psychological studies we used in our course showed that couples who experience infertility often go through a process of grieving for the children they cannot have that is as intense, and sometimes more enduring, than that of parents who suffer a stillbirth or loss of a newborn.[57] Some of this grief may be the result of socialization and hence susceptible to being addressed or eased by counseling. My co-panelist, Diane Aronson, headed a support group, Resolve, that is dedicated to helping infertile couples identify various ways of coping with the fact of infertility, from the use of infertility procedures to adoption or the emotional acceptance of childlessness. But women's persistence in trying cycles of IVF, often long after their doctors counsel stopping, is testimony to the power of the desire to have children of one's own, whatever the reason.

If these facts are reasonably clear to anyone who has studied infertility, why do so many Americans regard it as of little importance or as a purely discretionary part of medicine, on a par with face-lifts or liposuction? There are probably many answers to this question, including the influence of centuries-old religious teachings that barrenness is a punishment from God. But the most basic reason for this relative indifference to a major disease category is that infertility is few people's problem. The great majority of adults have either already had children or have chosen not to have any. Those who are busy coping with the many challenges of parenthood are usually unconcerned with the problem of childlessness. Unlike other well-researched disease conditions like cancer, heart disease, and neurological disorders, which threaten everyone no matter what their age, infertility is a problem that most mature people have left behind. This leaves only younger people, including the undergraduates I teach. For very different reasons, they, too, are unconcerned. Often involved in their very first sexual encounters, many are struggling with the opposite problem: how to avoid becoming parents before they want to. This leaves a substantial minority, the estimated one-tenth to one-twelfth of the population who experience infertility during their lives.[58] Poorly organized, isolated from one another, and silenced by embarrassment or shame, they are not in a position to educate society at large about the dimensions of their suffering.

As Van Blerkom wound up his testimony, it struck me that a large part of the problem behind the poor research he described is traceable to this generalized ignorance about infertility. Many progressive individuals who hold no particular religious or ideological presuppositions see little reason to spend scarce federal funds on a research agenda that does not seem to be of pressing importance. Some believe that adoption is an adequate solution to the problem. This ignores the fact that adoption often involves more obstacles and problems than does assisted reproduction, and that many people, fertile and infertile, regard themselves as unsuited to be adoptive parents.[59] Others believe that infertility is a problem only of well-to-do individuals who can afford their own care and research.[60] It is true that, as a group, white women are much more likely than Hispanic or African American women to utilize infertility services.[61] This reflects their generally higher economic status. Nevertheless, the experience of infertility is not confined to class or race. In fact, infertility occurs more frequently among African American than white couples.[62]

As a result of all these attitudes, relatively few active, middle-of-the-road supporters exist for government spending in this area. New initiatives and research are easily blocked by well-organized "pro-life" interest groups opposed to any forms of reproductive research. This combination of indifference and opposition is one cause of the fifteen-year-long *de facto* moratorium on embryo research.

At issue is nothing less than reproductive freedom. Over the course of my adult life, I have watched with satisfaction as the courts have come to understand this freedom as one of the basic liberties implied in the U.S. Constitution. In a host of decisions, courts have affirmed the basic legal right to make one's own family-related and reproductive decisions unimpeded by all but the most pressing state interests. As early as 1942, in the landmark decision *Skinner* v. *Oklahoma*, the Supreme Court affirmed the right to reproduce as one of "the basic civil rights of man."[63] In the 1965 decision *Griswold* v. *Connecticut*, the Supreme Court extended this tradition by upholding a couple's right *not* to have a child against their will when it struck down state laws preventing access to birth control methods.[64] In *Roe* v. *Wade* (1973), a right to privacy was interpreted to extend to a freedom from state intrusion in the decision to terminate a pregnancy.[65] Although the matter has not yet worked its way up to the Supreme Court, at least one lower court decision[66] and some theorists have suggested that the same right of reproductive freedom would apply to the protection of citizens' right not to have the government interfere with their efforts to have a child by means of assisted reproductive technologies.[67]

Of course, the moral and legal right not to be legally barred in one's pursuit of parenthood does not establish a corresponding claim on the government to support research or other means to this goal. Philosophers have distinguished between negative and positive rights. The former is the right not to be obstructed by others in one's exercise of some freedom; the latter involves the provision by the state or society of resources—educational opportunities, legal defense, or forms of health care—that are needed to pursue one's goals.[68]

U.S. law is far more inclined to recognize negative rather than positive rights. The developing constitutional tradition of reproductive liberty has largely focused on freedom from intervention by the government in reproductive decisions. Despite this history, a strong case can be made that if couples are free to use these new technologies, the government has the obligation at least to support research on their safety and efficacy. The government already spends billions of dollars each year through the NIH and other agencies on basic and applied health research aimed at improving understanding and treatment of a host of disease conditions. The best-known of the NIH institutes, such as the National Cancer Institute and the National Institute for Heart, Lung and Blood, address widespread, severe diseases. Other institutes deal with less threatening, but nonetheless distressing, medical problems experienced by small numbers of citizens. The National Institute for Deafness and Communication Disorders is one example. Few people die as a result of hearing problems or stuttering, yet millions of dollars are spent annually researching these and similar problems. Why should infertility be treated differently? Although it may be true that people have no positive right to assistance with their infertility, their negative right to governmental nonobstruction certainly implies a right of equitable treatment in the use of federal funds. As citizens whose taxes pay for research into a host of disease conditions suffered by others, why should infertile people's health problems be ignored?

This neglect becomes even more unfair and discriminatory when it is understood as stemming in part from organized opposition by religious groups. Imagine how society would react if federal funding for speech disorders were opposed by groups who believed that muteness is a divinely imposed punishment undeserving of a medical response? How would we feel if Jehovah's Witnesses blocked research on the safety of the blood supply because of their religiously based opposition to transfusions? The parallels to the religious opposition to embryo research are not complete, but they are suggestive. Would not such opposition raise issues of constitutional importance? I will return to this issue in my conclusion, when I look directly at how we are to assess the now decades-long obstruction of embryo research by organized religious groups.

Regardless of whether infertility procedures merit research aimed at their improvement, no one can dispute the fact that inadequate research in this area currently imposes real health risks on women and children. Infertility medicine is now being practiced in more than 350 clinics around the country. In view of our legal and ethical respect for reproductive liberty, these efforts will surely continue. As a result, each year thousands of women are subjected to powerful drugs with unknown consequences for long-term health, and thousands of children are born, some of whom are injured by poorly understood procedures. Certainly, the mandate of federal health research extends to protecting these people. A further consequence of the absence of a federal presence in this area is that research goes on without the oversight provided by federal human subjects regulations.[69] As I thought about all these matters, it became clearer to me why administrators at the National Institute of Child Health & Human Development were at the forefront of those at the NIH who wanted to see our panel formed.

That first day's meeting ended with a series of brief public statements that reinforced many things I was thinking but also signaled some of the problems that lay ahead. Because we were a public panel acting under the provisions of the Federal Advisory Committee Act, we were required to keep all meetings and communications open to the public. NIH staffers published notices of our meetings in the Federal Register and had written 240 letters to organizations with interests in the issue, inviting them to submit written statements to the panel or sign up, on a first-come, first-served basis, to deliver oral presentations. In the closing hour of the day we heard from several of these speakers.

Testimony by Dr. Maria Bustillo, a reproductive endocrinologist at Mt. Sinai Hospital, amplified Van Blerkom's comments. Dr. Bustillo spoke as a member of the board of directors of the Society for Assisted Reproduction (SART), the organization representing the research interests of infertility programs across the country, and as a member of the board of the Society for the Advancement of Women's Health Research. She began by noting the negative impact of the absence of federal funding on research in reproductive medicine. Most breakthroughs in this area were taking place outside the United States, she observed. After emphasizing how research might improve understanding of infertility and pregnancy loss, she went on to offer a wider picture. Better understanding of cellular differentiation in the early embryo might shed light on the origins of certain genetic diseases[70] and pediatric and other cancers. Closer study of the process of embryo development, embryogenesis, might help us understand how toxins, maternal nutritional deficiencies, infectious diseases, and other factors lead to fetal death and serious birth defects. A better understanding of fertilization and embryo implantation might enhance control of these processes, leading to safer and more effective contraceptives.

I found the last point to be particularly interesting. As a teacher of ethics, I have repeatedly reminded students that in assessing the consequences of a decision, they should be prepared for paradox. Real causal connections in the world are frequently the *opposite* of what one might expect, and one must take this "perversity of reality" into account in morally assessing a practice or policy. A familiar example is laws that require health care professionals to report drug abuse by pregnant women. These well-intentioned laws aim at protecting the fetus or newborn, but they frequently have just the opposite effect. Because many drug-abusing pregnant women fear exposure or arrest, these laws can cause them to avoid the health care system entirely.[71] This defeats the laws' purpose of identifying drug-abusing mothers and deprives these women and their children of basic care.

Bustillo's observation about the link between infertility research and improved contraception provided another example of the importance of understanding real causal links as we make moral and policy judgments. One of the most common criticisms of infertility medicine, and of any research aimed at improving it, is that these efforts hardly seem to be needed in a world already bursting at the seams with people. Our problems are overpopulation and environmental degradation, not infertility. What Bustillo's remarks showed, however, is that, paradoxically, the causal links here may be much more complex than we think. Infertility research can lead to population reduction. Throughout the world, a major contributing factor to the population problem is the lack of good contraceptive methods. Barrier methods—condoms, diaphragms, and foams—have high failure rates and are not well accepted by many people. Current birth control pills not only have health consequences that make them objectionable to many women, they are also subject to failure through forgetfulness and human error. At one point, the longer-acting implant Norplant looked like a promising alternative, but the need for skilled personnel for its insertion and removal and the drug's side effects have made it a source of controversy.[72]

If infertility research has shown one thing, however, it is that fertilization and implantation are very complex processes that can go wrong in many ways. The failure of a single chemical signal can block fertilization or lead a fertilized embryo to pass out of a woman's reproductive tract without implanting. The purpose of infertility research is to correct this kind of problem, but, applied in the other direction, the knowledge gained from this research can also lead to new, more effective ways of preventing pregnancies. Imagine, for example, the implications of finding, as some evidence already suggests, that a major cause of infertility is a woman's immune response to her partner's sperm. In the future, understanding this might lead to a simple vaccine that could provide months or years of reversible contraception. Understanding what is needed for the sperm to penetrate the egg might make possible a simple post-coital suppository to prevent fertilization. Better research might even enhance the efficacy of the rhythm method, the one form of contraception permitted by the Roman Catholic church. Paradoxically, therefore, infertility research may make a major contribution to reducing the population problem. The relatively small number of children brought into being by these technologies would be dwarfed by massive reductions in birth rates as new forms of contraception allowed couples to maintain their desired family size. A deeper lesson here, of course, is that the best human response to a problem always lies in enhancing research and knowledge, not perpetuating ignorance. By increasing the range of choices for infertile couples, infertility medicine makes possible greater choice for those who wish to control the size of their families. In this regard, reproductive freedom is of one piece. Respect for the right to have children enhances one's right *not* to have them.

The remainder of the public testimony that afternoon fell into opposing camps. Two individuals addressed the panel about their experiences of infertility and expressed strong support for research. One of these, Rick Sellers, happily reported that he was the father of a three-week-old baby born as a result of assisted reproductive technology. He discussed the emotional suffering he and his wife had gone through in their efforts to have a child, and he criticized what he called the "insidious discrimination" that deprived reproductive system disorders of the moral, legal, and social attention accorded to other ailments. Both he and a second presenter from the infertility perspective, Jolene Hall Slotter, reported that they would be willing to donate to research any embryos remaining from their procedures. But they noted that their primary goal was having the children they wanted, and this placed a limit on their ability to donate eggs or embryos for research purposes.

In sharp opposition to this view was the testimony of two Roman Catholic spokesmen, William E. May from the Pope John XXIII Medical Moral Research Center, a Roman Catholic bioethics "think tank" in Massachusetts,[73] and Richard Doerflinger, associate director of the leading Roman Catholic political action office in the area of abortion, the Secretariat for Pro-Life Activities of the National Conference of Catholic Bishops. Looking back, I can now see the irony in the fact that these two speakers had almost the last word that day. Months later, they also had the last word on the work of our panel. If this narrative has a villain, it is Richard Doerflinger. I say this not to impugn his integrity or character. In fact, Doerflinger is a dedicated and zealous proponent of his church's views. He does his job very well, and, on a personal level, we get along well. Nevertheless, despite his obvious intelligence, not once throughout the year did his published writings, statements, or personal remarks to me evidence any willingness to understand the case for embryo research or enter into real dialogue about what might be good public policy in this area. The Roman Catholic church opposes nontherapeutic manipulations of the human embryo, that is, manipulations not of direct benefit for the embryo under study.[74] That message would be sent out to the Catholic faithful who, in turn, would be asked to return it, in thousands of postcards and letters, to our panel, to the NIH, and, above all, to Congress.

Doerflinger began combatively. The panel, he said, was "a special interest group" whose members "have financial or other personal interests" in pursuing embryo research. This theme, animated by attacks on the motives and character of each member of the panel, became a leitmotif of Doerflinger's articles in the Roman Catholic press throughout the year.[75] Although it was probably useful as a strategy for undermining the panel's credibility in the minds of those remote from the issues, it also unfairly represented the whole process of expert review of complex biomedical issues. But fairness was not high on Doerflinger's agenda. As far as substance was concerned, he had one message: the embryo is a fully human subject from the time of conception. The burden of proof rests on those who believe that federal human subjects regulations should treat it differently before implantation than after implantation. In response to a question from Carol Tauer about whether nonviable embryos remaining from infertility procedures, embryos otherwise destined to be destroyed, might be used for research, Doerflinger had a succinct reply: they are dying human subjects. Research on them (including, presumably, research using the polyploid or radically defective embryos sometimes encountered in infertility medicine) is just like using a dying AIDS victim in an experiment without that individual's consent.

This equation of the early embryo with adult patients was central to Doerflinger's message. Earlier that day, Van Blerkom's had shown many slides of embryos, now the subject of Doerflinger's testimony. Although I realize that an intensive effort at moral reasoning might lead someone to regard this entity as a human being, Doerflinger's quick response to Carol's question emphasized the evident leap he was asking us to make. We were being told that a microscopic ball of cells whose chromosomes were so abnormal that it could not develop any further is morally equivalent to a dying AIDS patient. What kind of thinking, I wondered, led to such detachment from reality?

May's testimony immediately preceded Doerflinger's and sounded many of the same themes. He affirmed the "incomparable dignity" of all members of the human species from the moment of conception. He reminded us of the

Nuremberg trials and the lessons they held for those who would abuse innocent persons for research goals. Although he was sympathetic with the plight
of infertile couples, he did not believe that IVF was an appropriate response
to the problem. It involved, he said, an improper use of medicine because it
merely satisfied couples' desires for children without "curing" their underlying infertility. Alta Charo, a law professor from the University of Wisconsin
who had little tolerance for sloppy arguments, quickly attacked this. She
asked May whether his prescription eyeglasses did not therefore constitute an
improper use of medicine, since they merely fulfilled his desire for better
vision without curing his underlying myopia. Refusing to retreat from his
opposition to IVF, May replied that he was in favor of surgical reconstruction
of blocked oviducts.[76]

As I listened to May speak, I recalled a question Van Blerkom had asked
earlier that day: "When does an embryo exist?" Van Blerkom pointed to the
fact that conception (or fertilization) itself requires definition. At what point
can we say that we are no longer dealing with two sex cells (an egg and a
sperm), but a human embryo? In trying to answer his own question, Van
Blerkom emphasized "syngamy," the coming together of the male and female
sets of chromosomes inside the egg. This usually happens eighteen to twenty-
six hours after the sperm first penetrates the egg's outer membrane. Van
Blerkom observed that syngamy sometimes does not occur despite the fact
that the sperm has penetrated the egg. In such cases, he said, one cannot
really say that the egg has been fertilized or that an embryo exists. Because
May and others who share his views place so much weight on conception, or
fertilization, as the starting point for the human person, I was curious to know
how he or his institute defined it.

"Dr. May," I began, "we have heard statements today from Dr. Van
Blerkom and others that, in fact, the process of fertilization is precisely that, a
process, that there is at least a substantial period of time between penetration
of the egg and syngamy. Does your group have a position with regard to the
moral status of the entity between penetration and syngamy?"

May's response was interesting. "I don't want to address the precise question of syngamy," he replied. "Certainly there is a process that takes place,
but there is some point at which fertilization/conception occurs. From that
point on, you do have a member of the human species." May then reiterated
his contention that life begins at fertilization/conception and added that this
takes place "not necessarily when the sperm first penetrates the ovum, but
when you have a zygote."[77] He did not further define what he meant by
zygote, although in standard medical parlance this refers to the single-cell
entity resulting from fertilization.

May's answer was curious. First, it was largely a nonanswer. Asked when
conception, or fertilization, occurs, he replied "when you have a zygote" but

never answered the further question of when this happens. The idea that it did not necessarily occur when the sperm penetrated the egg was helpful, but no answer was offered to the next question, whether syngamy was the decisive event. More curious was the lack of precision on this point. Here was a question that would be crucial for us to answer if we accepted the view that conception, or fertilization, had the significance that May and Doerflinger said it did. Yet May, a representative of one of the leading Roman Catholic research centers dedicated to thinking about ethical issues dealing with reproduction, was unable to furnish an expert panel with any opinion on this point. In defense of his imprecision, one could say that these were novel matters that we all were just beginning to examine. Historically, one also could point to the fact that the Roman Catholic church often takes positions on broad ethical issues without waiting for all the scientific or definitional details to be nailed down. The church's general opposition to active euthanasia, for example, has not depended on a precise definition of death, which is still under consideration.[78]

Nevertheless, I found May's imprecision startling. It suggested to me that he and his associates, like many people, had not really thought about the question at all.[79] There was a "moment" of conception, and that was that. In fact, Van Blerkom had already made it clear that there is not just one self-evident event that marks the transformation from sex cell to zygote, but separate candidate events (sperm penetration, syngamy, perhaps others) separated in time and occurring over a period of time. Like all biological occurrences, in other words, even something that seems so all-or-nothing, so "on or off" as conception involves certain processes. This means that in understanding these processes and incorporating them into our ethical and political thinking, we must always decide *which* events in the sequence, or *which* magnitudes of change, are significant and which are not.

In the next chapter, when I review the thinking that underlay my specific contributions to the panel's work, I will return to this matter at length. For now, I want only to say that May's response to my question indicated that these ideas were utterly alien to him. Nothing in the biological realm required decisions on our part. All we need to do is read information and instructions off the book of nature. God (who in matters as ethically important as this surely would not leave us without explicit guidance) had written that book. If life begins at conception, as May and Doerflinger unhesitatingly affirmed, then conception must be something obvious. It would be nice if this were true. But our increasing understanding of biology does not support it. May's approach thus became a way of avoiding the questions, or even of imposing his own set of answers to them on everyone else.

I may be wrong about all this. Perhaps May's thinking was more sophisticated than our brief encounter suggested. But certainly this way of thinking is widely prevalent in our society. Many people continue to believe that there are clear, indisputable biological markers "out there" that compel our judgment about life's beginning. In the next chapter I will speculate as to why this way of thinking remains so prevalent, and I will suggest that it sometimes influences even fairly sophisticated scientists and philosophers.

If the first day of our first meeting enhanced our understanding of the importance of our work and the challenges we faced, the second day, 3 February, left us with a sense that in some key areas that called for reflection, we were on our own. The day featured two presentations, each of which, in different ways, left us with more questions than answers. Lori Andrews, a health care lawyer from the Kent-Chicago College of Law, began the morning with comments on a paper that she had prepared that reviewed existing statutory and case law on issues related to embryo research. As she spoke, I recalled the old joke about the recently arrested mobster who tells the policeman at the jailhouse that he wants a one-handed lawyer. "One-handed? Why?," the policeman asks. The mobster replies, "All the lawyers I meet say, 'On the one hand, you can do this; on the other hand, you can do that.' I want a lawyer who'll tell me what to do."

Andrews was not equivocal, but the excellent overview of legal issues she provided us was.[80] We learned that other nations are clearly divided on this issue. A survey of eleven countries revealed that one (Norway) prohibits human embryo research outright; six (Australia, Austria, Denmark, France, Germany, and Switzerland) allow research, but only under very limited conditions; and four (Canada, Spain, Sweden, and the United Kingdom) liberally permit research. Of these four, the United Kingdom's regulations, supervised by the HFEA, are the least restrictive and include the freedom to create embryos for research.[81] In the United States, a small number of states have laws banning most embryo research. Louisiana's law is probably the most restrictive. It regards the early embryo as a juridical person meriting all the protections given children or adult research subjects.[82] Andrews reported that a justice of the Louisiana Supreme Court had told her that this law was a "Trojan horse" designed to force a reconsideration of women's abortion rights. If embryo research could be banned, then so might other activities that put the embryo or fetus at risk.

Apart from these few clear state laws, which might not hold up on constitutional review, we learned that there is little in U.S. law to guide our thinking. Behind us lay a broad constitutional acceptance of reproductive freedom and freedom of scientific research. Ahead lay no clear legal or constitutional guidelines concerning what a panel like ours might recommend. As far as U.S. law was concerned, we were on our own, with future legal initiatives and rulings likely to support or undermine our efforts.

The final presenter that day was Bonnie Steinbock, a bioethicist from the

State University of New York at Albany. She had prepared a long paper for our review and was present to offer comments on it.[83] The focus of her remarks was on a question that she deemed "absolutely crucial" for our work: the moral status of the human embryo. "Whether the human embryo is perceived as a human being or a human subject would determine what kinds of research, if any, it may be used in," she observed. If the human embryo were to be regarded as a fully human subject, like any adult or pediatric patient, then research would be severely limited. Only procedures promising therapeutic benefit for the embryo (or at most, minimal risks to its healthy survival) would be permitted. If it had lesser claims, then research that ended in the destruction of the embryo but benefited others or increased scientific knowledge might be allowed.

I had long been professionally interested in the question of how we determine the moral status and claims of humans and other beings. I was acquainted with Steinbock's writings, and, for me at least, her presentation covered familiar ground. She began by drawing on the abortion debate to identify three broad approaches to the issue. "Conservatives" on abortion, she said, take the position that embryos are human subjects because they are genetically human. This is all that it is needed to establish its basic claim to full moral respect. Some who share this view also stress the fact that embryos have the natural potential to develop into children. Unless actively interfered with, an embryo in the womb will become a child. Although this idea of natural potential makes sense when applied to most embryos, she noted, it may have less force in the context of reproductive medicine, where the embryo cannot possibly progress without massive assistance from medical specialists.

At the other end of the spectrum of views, she continued, are "liberals," who believe that "humanity" is a moral concept. According to this view, when we ask the question, "Is this entity human?" we are not merely seeking biological information but are trying to determine whether it possesses sacredness, the inherent right to life, and all the other protections we normally associate with human beings. To distinguish the biological from this moral (or legal) use of the term "human," and to avoid foreclosing our answer to these questions, philosophers had introduced the question of whether a human being is a "person."[84] Thus, an anencephalic baby born with little or no brain matter (on clinical rounds I have seen anencephalic babies whose brain cavity contained only clear fluid) is *human* in a genetic sense. So, too, is the patient whose neocortex has been destroyed as a result of a massive stroke or injury, but whose lower brain stem maintains heart function. But many people would argue that neither of these is *morally* a human being, a "person," whom we should fight to keep alive.

What is it, then, that makes something a "person"? If it is not just a question of genetic or biological humanity, which qualities are determinative? Addressing this question, Steinbock indicated that those holding this position usually point to a range of cognitive capacities, such as the ability to reason, to communicate, to use language, and to become a moral agent. Steinbock acknowledged holding a variation of this position herself, which she called the "interest view." According to this, the minimum requirement for having an interest is sentience, the ability to feel pain. The interest view, she affirmed, is somewhat broader than other "personhood" views because it accords respect to newborn infants and the mentally retarded. It also establishes a degree of moral status for animals. But it does not find even the minimal basis for moral respect in early embryos because, not yet having developed the tissues or organs needed for sentience, they have no "interests."

A third position, said Steinbock, represents something of a compromise between these extremes. Although it is like the liberal views in denying that the embryo is a human being in a moral sense, it sees it as a developing form of human life that possesses "symbolic value." This symbolic value provides the basis for careful restrictions on the nature and extent of embryo research. Steinbock pointed out that virtually every national commission that has investigated the subject has taken this third position. Although neither she nor any of us listening could know it at the time, this was close to the position our panel would take.

Steinbock's presentation was more or less a textbook philosophical introduction to the topic. The distinction between biological humanity and moral personhood was essential. So, too, was the range of views she sketched. Yet, as I listened to her, I became aware of my discomfort with this standard approach to the issue. Where the early embryo is concerned, we are dealing with an entity that in some respects upsets all our accustomed ways of thinking. The preimplantation embryo presents a variety of challenges to those who believe that the presence of genetic humanity is a sufficient answer to our questions. It raises the question of what we mean by genetic identity, both at the beginning of the embryo's development, when it resides in a borderland between gamete and zygote, and throughout the earliest phases of its development, when each of its cells, or "blastomeres," retains the ability to develop into a complete human being. As Steinbock herself realized, potentiality arguments also become odd in this highly technologized reproductive context.

Those on the "left" avoid these biological problems by emphasizing developed cognitive abilities, but they face problems of their own. Why is the ability to reason or use language so decisive? Where do these criteria come from, and how do we know they are the right ones? Why is having "interests" the key issue, as Steinbock argued, and why is sentience important to this determination? Steinbock told us that animals, because they are sentient, have moral status, "although not necessarily the same moral status as human persons." How does she know this? Who decides how much sentience is needed for moral status? Listening to her report of the arguments from the right and the left, I knew that something fundamental was being left out: an explicit discussion of how we think about these criteria in the first place. The important first question, I noted, is not *which* qualities or properties makes something morally human, but *how* we know what those qualities or properties are.

In the course of my work, I had a spent a great deal of time thinking about this more basic question. I hoped that I would eventually be able to make a contribution to the panel by bringing some of this thinking to bear on our work. As I was considering what contribution I could make, the question suddenly ceased being speculative. Drawing the meeting to a close, our chair, Steven Muller, who had earlier described himself as the nonspecialist "ringmaster" of our efforts, suggested that as early as the next meeting in March it would be useful to have drafts of our report's most important chapters. Brigid Hogan volunteered to work on an introductory chapter on the scientific issues. Pat King agreed to orchestrate work on the draft of a chapter dealing with some of the leading ethical and policy issues. In connection with Pat's work, I was asked to put together a brief document reviewing the positions we might take on the moral status of the human embryo. Bernard Lo was asked to prepare an overview of alternatives for assessing and regulating gamete or embryo donation for research, and Carol Tauer would review the matter of possible time limits on research. Suddenly, as our first two-day meeting ended, I found myself charged with helping to shape our thinking on what Bonnie Steinbock had earlier called the most "crucial" question before the panel.

2

DETERMINING MORAL STATUS

THE panel's next meeting was slated for 14 March. This meant that those of us who were assigned writing responsibilities had a little more than a month to prepare documents that would greatly shape the panel's work. My assignment was to review alternatives and develop the outlines of a position on the moral status of the embryo, one of the most controversial issues facing the panel and our society as a whole. Returning to Dartmouth, I mentioned this assignment to a colleague. "When you finish this," she quipped, "why don't you take another month and write a chapter on the meaning of life."

The challenge of determining the moral status of the human embryo was sharpened by the public context in which our panel was working. This was not just a matter of an ethicist sitting in an armchair trying to arrive at the most persuasive view of the matter. The panel's recommendations would affect the direction of public policy and the spending of public funds. Many people in our society hold strong views on the embryo's status. The question, therefore, was not just which view is the most compelling, but which one should form the basis of governmental conduct in a pluralistic society in which people hold very different views on the issue. To the usual requirement that one's arguments be good, I had to add attention to the larger political and social ramifications of any position we took.

A first task was to review my own thinking about how we establish the moral status of an entity or, what is the same, the degree of moral protection it should receive. This question arises in a variety of contexts. We meet it in discussions about our moral obligations to animals. We also encounter it at the end of life, when we must determine whether an individual whose physical condition has greatly deteriorated still merits aggressive efforts at treatment. But the question is found in its most difficult form in discussions of the status of the developing human embryo. Here, it is often put in terms of when the embryo becomes "a human being," or when "human life" in a moral sense is thought to begin. Over the years I had written about these questions in the context of the abortion debate.[85] I would now try to bring that thinking to bear on the status of the early human embryo.

I believe that I had two key insights to offer on this matter. One is the understanding that biological occurrences are processes rather than events. Nature rarely, if ever, presents definitive transitions from one state of being to another. Instead, elements within a biological system undergo continuous change. At some observable points transitions occur, but the importance or discreteness of these apparent "events" is usually a function of the precision of our measuring instruments. In an era in which we can track changes at microscopic levels and in milliseconds of time, "events" that used to seem almost instantaneous, like a cell's division, now appear as complex and extended processes with many discrete and ever-changing components.

This first insight leads to a second. Because biological realities involve processes, the determination of significant points within these processes inevitably involves choice and decision on our part. This means that our conclusions are never dictated merely by the discovery of important features or states in an entity. Rather, identifying these features or states requires us to ask why this region on the curve of transition is important to us, or why we want to describe a particular magnitude of change as a decisive "event." This is true not only for matters of scientific description, but also for matters that involve moral issues. In selecting a point on the curve of biological change as one that should alter our moral practice, we are making a decision. This, in turn, forces us to examine the purposes and values that shape that decision. In an earlier writing, I described this insight as representing a "Copernican revolution" in our thinking about ethical issues related to the life sciences.[86] Copernicus changed our view of the earth from one that saw it as the passive center of the universe to one that sees it as an active, moving object. Similarly, the insight that our values lead us to select morally significant points on the curve of otherwise continuous biological processes converts us from passive identifiers of biologically fixed truths to active choosers of markers on life's spectrum.

These points are abstract, but they become more concrete when one turns to what is known and being learned about the early human embryo. The problem is first encountered when we try to determine at what point the embryo can even be said to exist. As Jonathan Van Blerkom told us, the answer is marked by uncertainty. Some believe that the embryo exists at the moment that the sperm comes into contact with the egg. At that time, they reason, two separate sex cells cease to be and the embryo (or zygote) begins to develop. But what does "contact" mean here? It has recently been found that the egg emits chemical signals that serve to attract sperm when the sperm are still relatively far off in the uterus and even before they have entered the fallopian tubes.[87] Do these "chemoattractant" signals amount to "contact"?

A better candidate for the fertilization "event," and, hence, the "beginning" of the embryo, might be the penetration of the egg's tough outer membrane (zona pellucida) by the sperm. This triggers a host of chemical changes that cause the sperm to undergo what is known as the "acrosome reaction."[88] At this time the genetic package carried in the sperm's head separates from the remainder of the cell body and passes through the zona into the egg's cytoplasm. This sets off a cascade of electrochemical reactions that are now being closely studied by reproductive biologists. Within seconds, signals pass to the zona that normally render it impenetrable by other sperm. If we think of fertilization as the beginning of a unique individual, the acrosome reaction might be a good candidate event, because from this time onward the product of conception usually results from only one sperm and one egg. But things are not quite that simple. Sometimes more than one sperm penetrates the egg, which results in polyploidy, an excess number of chromosomes in the zygote.[89] Although this condition usually prevents further development or results in stillbirth, sometimes the embryo is able to correct the problem by ejecting the excess chromosomes. This highlights the fact that the new diploid genome remains unstable for a considerable period of time after sperm penetration of the egg. Should we perhaps say that fertilization has occurred only after all these possibilities have been eliminated?

Or should we stipulate that fertilization occurs at an even later time? Once inside the egg, the remaining parts of the sperm trigger further events. The egg itself now completes sexual division. It extrudes half of its forty-six chromosomes to form a "polar body," a small sphere adjacent to the egg proper.[90] The egg's remaining twenty-three chromosomes migrate to the cell's center, where, eighteen to twenty-six hours later, they line up with the twenty-three chromosomes from the sperm. This is syngamy, literally, the "spouses joining together." In biological terms, if we think of a new individual as coming into being with the appearance of a cell having a new "diploid" genome, a full complement of forty-six chromosomes, syngamy would seem to be a good candidate for a starting point. This is the moment that the "zygote" is said to come into being. Some legal jurisdictions that ban embryo research and that must therefore define when the embryo comes into being have chosen syn-gamy as the defining event.[91]

However, there are some problems with viewing syngamy as decisive. Biol-ogists usually describe the cells of an organism as having the full range of cellular structures, including a single cell nucleus that contains DNA within its own nuclear membrane. But at syngamy the zygote has no definitive nu-clear membrane. Up to this point, the genetic material is contained in the two "pronuclei" of the male and female gametes that have begun to break down and blend together.[92] A distinctive diploid cell nucleus does not make its ap-pearance until the two-cell stage, after the zygote undergoes its first cell divi-sion, which may occur anywhere from twenty-four to thirty-six hours after sperm penetration. Is the zygote, then, not the start of the embryo? Must we await the appearance of a two-cell entity following the first cleavage division?[93]

Further complicating matters is the fact that the twenty-three paternal chromosomes apparently do no work at all during the first few cell divisions. In human beings, the earliest developmental process, at least until the eight-cell stage, seems to be entirely governed by egg cell structures and the mater-nal chromosomes.[94] This is why a parthenote (or parthenogenote), an egg that has never been fertilized but that has been stimulated electrically or chem-ically, can be made to cleave for several divisions. During the earliest phase of its development, when only maternal chromosomes are active, the parthenote looks and behaves exactly like an embryo, although in humans its growth inevitably stops at the four- or eight-cell stage, when the presence of paternal genetic material is needed for further development. In human beings, a working set of forty-six chromosomes is necessary for new human cells to exist, but such chromosomes do not appear until the four- or eight-cell stage of development. Thus, we have a number of equally compelling candidate events for the start of an embryo, events spread out over a period of perhaps twenty-four to forty-eight hours. This indicates how misleading it is to speak of "the moment of fertilization." Instead, as one recent embryology textbook puts it, "fertilization is a series of processes rather than a single event."[95]

"All right," one may respond, "fertilization is a process, but once it is com-plete at twenty-four or forty-eight hours and we have a tiny developing em-bryo, then we can affirm with certainty that we have the start of a new human individual." Unfortunately, many odd features of the early embryo challenge this view. During the initial phases of cell division, and usually beyond the point when it is returned to the womb in current IVF procedures, many of the embryo's individual cells, or blastomeres, remain "totipotent." That is, each blastomere is undifferentiated and remains capable, if properly manipu-lated, of developing into a full human being. In 1993, a George Washington University research team made headlines by exploiting this feature of the early embryo.[96] They took chromosomally defective (triploid) embryos left over from infertility procedures, split them in two, and provided the cluster of blastomeres composing each half with a protective artificial zona pellucida made of agar gel. The embryos went on to cleave and grow just as though they had never been split. There is good reason to believe that, if the embryos had been chromosomally normal and if the researchers had placed them back in a womb, some would have gone on to produce healthy babies. Embryo splitting of this sort—or blastomere separation, as it is technically called—has already been performed successfully in other species, including cows.[97] The George Washington University team's efforts were aimed at multiplying the number of embryos available to infertile couples for reproductive purposes. In a kind of "loaves and fishes" way, they hoped that one embryo could become two, cleave, then become four, eight, and so on. Their work generated controversy because it is a form of cloning, theoretically permitting the mass replication of genotypes in a manner not unlike the "Bokanovsky process" depicted in *Brave New World*.[98] Unfortunately for reproductive medicine, no evidence exists that any net gain for couples can be accomplished by these methods because the survivability of the individual embryos seems to decline proportionally as their numbers increase.

This splitting of the early embryo is not limited to research contexts. In nature, embryo splitting happens spontaneously in from two to five out of every 1000 human births.[99] The result is identical (monozygotic) twins, triplets, or higher-order multiples. If biological humanness starts with the appearance of a unique diploid genome, twins and triplets are living evidence that the early embryo is not yet one human being, but a community of possibly different individuals held together by a gelatinous membrane. In the words of a recent embryology text, during the first two postovulatory weeks "the production of a single individual versus multiple individuals is not yet irrevocable. . . . A genetically unique but non-individuated embryo has yet to acquire determinate individuality, a stable human identity."[100]

In nature, this possibility definitively comes to an end only at about fourteen days of development, with the beginning of gastrulation and the appearance of the primitive streak. Only at this point do all the cells of the embryonic disk lose their totipotency and become committed to specialized fates. By approximately one week after the start of gastrulation, a line of precursor neuronal cells has formed in the top cell layer of the primitive streak. These cells go on to become the brain and nervous system of the developing individual.

Because at least some embryonic cells of the inner cell mass remain totipotent until the formation of the primitive streak, perhaps it is the blastomere or its undifferentiated successor cells, rather than the embryo, that is the true human individual. But several considerations cast doubt on this idea. Are we to think of the early embryo's multiple totipotent cells as a community of many human individuals that somehow, in most (but not all) cases, eventually become one person? If so, what becomes of the missing "individuals"? Another problem is that many of the early blastomeres do not go on to produce a fetus but instead give rise to placental or other auxiliary tissues.[101] Also noteworthy is the fact that despite its potential for development, each blastomere is utterly dispensable. In normal embryogenesis, some blastomeres die, but the embryo nevertheless continues to grow normally. In preimplantation genetic diagnosis, a single blastomere is removed by microsurgery from the developing embryo and subjected to molecular analysis for genetic disorders. This loss of a blastomere in no way harms the embryo, which goes on to develop into a fetus.[102]

Another complicating factor for a blastomere-level view of human individuality is that in some cases, the frequency of which in the human population has not been precisely determined, separate and genetically distinct embryos (which might have gone on to become fraternal twins) fuse during early development to form a single human being.[103] When this happens, processes of intracellular signaling take over and all the cells receive instructions to perform their specialized roles in one body. This produces individuals known as chimeras, that have two or more cell lines scattered throughout their bodies from different fertilized eggs. When the cells involved have different pairs of sex chromosomes, the result can sometimes be hermaphroditism and the appearance of ambiguous genitalia. Genetically and physically, these people are literally part male and part female. Sometimes, however, chimerism occurs with very early embryos that have inherited the same pair of sex-determining chromosomes. The resulting individuals can go through their entire lives without realizing they are chimeras. Some show patches of different hair or skin coloring. Occasionally, a blood test may reveal the presence of cells with two distinct blood types. If one of these people undergoes genetic testing for a familial disorder, tests may reveal some cells with a mutation and others without it.

All of these properties of the early embryo and its component cells make it problematic to speak of the existence of a single biological individual at this time in development.[104] Taking these new biological perspectives into account, influential Roman Catholic thinkers like Norman Ford, Richard McCormick, and Thomas Shannon have asked whether, even on the narrowest biological grounds, the true beginning of the "individual human being" can be traced to fertilization.[105] Ford and McCormick both argue that the appearance of the primitive streak is a better candidate event than is fertilization. Having reached this point in development, each of the individual cells in the embryo is sufficiently differentiated that it can produce only bodily tissues, not a full human being.

Some object to the use of this information in this way. During the second day of the panel's meeting, Lori Andrews expressed puzzlement over the argument that the possibility of twinning reduces the moral claims of the very early embryo. Why manipulate or destroy any of these cells if they can lead to one or more human individuals in the future? "Should it matter that you can't predict how many entities you're going to harm?" she asked.[106] But this question misses the point. The issue here is whether the embryo, while still capable of becoming more (or less) than one being, really is an identifiable "individual" for either biological or moral purposes. This question is critical for those who believe that the appearance of the embryo at fertilization marks the beginning of a new "human individual" that merits some degree of moral protection. It is a question that can no more be ignored than the question of whether a sperm and egg, in the instant before their union, represent a single human being worthy of moral protection or merely two separate and morally insignificant gametes.

Roman Catholic theorists are particularly sensitive to this definitional problem. Catholic theology defines the human soul as "an individual substance of a rational nature."[107] The soul is an individual reality, and every human individual can have only one soul. Because the presence of the human soul is what makes a being morally sacred in Catholic thinking, this definition renders unavoidable the question of whether, from a Catholic perspective, a collection of blastomeres that can become more than one person can in any way be considered an ensouled human being. Wrestling with this question, Albert S. Moraczewski, a conservative Catholic thinker, has tried to preserve the idea that individual human life begins at fertilization/conception while acknowledging the biological reality of twinning. The individual "ensouled" person is the zygote that comes into being at conception, he argues. In the case of twinning, the zygote can be thought of as giving rise to its twin by means of asexual, clonal type reproduction.[108] But this solution not only introduces an odd new view of the human reproductive process, with siblings giving rise asexually to siblings, but it also renders fertilization a less decisive event for some individuals' beginnings. It also falters in the face of embryo fusion. What are we to say when blastomeres from one fertilization event, which might have gone on to become a person, join a cluster of other, genetically different blastomeres to become a new individual? Has the first "person's" soul vanished? Perhaps it is better to conclude that no "soul" is present at this time and that "ensoulment" occurs only with the appearance of the primitive streak, once the possibility of these twinning and fusion events comes to an end.[109]

I am by no means suggesting that we settle these matters by determining when the soul is present in early embryos. This is a metaphysical question pertaining to religious faith, not something that can be determined by the means available to those who must form public policy. I emphasize the special puzzles that these complex biological facts raise for traditional approaches because they bring to the fore the point I have been making. Biology does not admit of definitive events. Instead it almost always involves complex processes with many occurrences and transitions happening over periods of time. Fertilization illustrates this idea of a continuum very well. What used to seem so definitive, given our lack of intimate understanding of the process, no longer is so. The same is true of the process of biological individuation. To the layperson, the human individual "comes into being" when a unique genome, or "genetic blueprint," for the person is established at fertilization. But even "uniqueness" here is a relative thing on a continuum of occurrences moving toward increasing individuation. A large number of individuals with different genomes can result from the active biological system that is present in the fallopian tube (or petri dish) before a sperm meets the egg. Fertilization (whenever that is said to occur) reduces this number significantly. But twinning and fusion events suggest that, even well after the formation of the zygote, biological individuality is not yet firmly established. Only at gastrulation can we say that the lengthy biological process of individuation is complete.

The understanding that biology involves continuous processes rather than events applies to the end of life as well as its beginning. Not long ago we believed that death was an event. The individual moved instantly from the realm of the living to the realm of the dead. Usually, this was thought to occur when respiration ceased for even a few minutes. This arrest of breathing inevitably and almost simultaneously brought with it permanent cessation of all other bodily functions. Today, however, we know that death is a series of occurrences, a process rather than a single event.[110] Science and technology have allowed us to separate out many of its component parts. When someone stops breathing, we can put her on a respirator to maintain oxygenation of the blood. If the heart stops, a pump can maintain circulation. Regions of the brain can cease functioning at different times, and some can be maintained while others begin to deteriorate. This raises the question of which aspects of this complex and extended process are morally significant. When should we say that something important enough has happened to allow us to conclude, a person has died?

Understanding that biological occurrences are processes leads us back to the second key insight I mentioned as relevant to thinking about questions of moral status and life's moral boundaries. Determination of morally significant points within these processes inevitably involves choices and decisions. It is not just a matter of *discovering* important events in the entity that must dictate our judgment. Rather, identifying these events requires us to identify and apply the values that underlie our thinking. Drawing on these values, we must *decide* which events are most important to us among the range of alternatives.

Because I have introduced the subject of death, let me illustrate this point with regard to the dying process. When the introduction of mechanical respirators made it clear to us that we could sustain respiration and circulation indefinitely in the absence of brain function, we suddenly became aware that we had to choose which functions of these various biological systems are morally important to us. Is anything of value achieved, we asked, by indefinitely sustaining a patient in a persistent vegetative state who will never regain consciousness and whose other biological systems are maintained by machines? Is the ability to sustain respiration and circulation without the possibility of consciousness important? Most people decided that it is not, and most legal jurisdictions have chosen the cessation of brain activity as a criterion of death.[111] In a different direction, when kidney dialysis became available and it became possible to sustain indefinitely those whose kidneys had failed, we had to determine how to respond to this new situation. Quickly, and almost unreflectively, we concluded that kidney functioning is not especially important to our understanding of the worth of human life. We barely even paused to consider the cessation of kidney function as indicating death. Instead, we committed ourselves to the long-term care of people whose kidneys fail. In different ways, these events illustrate how value-based choices underlie our thinking about what counts as determining the occurrence of death.[112]

I realize that it seems odd to describe the determination of when death occurs as a matter of choice. If anything seems to be "out there," a state we merely identify or discover, death is it. But there are reasons why we react in this way. In the past, two factors worked together to obscure our understanding of the choice-based nature of our approach to life's moral boundaries. One was a rudimentary level of technological advance, and the other was a habit of mind shaped by religious ways of thinking.

Limited or rudimentary technology narrowed our range of choices. In doing so, it contributed to the view that identifying death involves no choice at all. Hard biological facts drove us toward only one conclusion. For example, until very recently, the definitive loss of spontaneous functioning by almost any single major organ system meant the rapid cessation of all other systems. Respiration, the one activity the cessation of which we could easily observe, was particularly important. When breathing stopped for a short period of time, the person was dead. There was nothing to "decide."

Despite the fact that we no longer take the cessation of spontaneous respiration as signifying death, technological limitations still make death appear to be an objectively determinable event independent of any decisions on our part. For example, it is common today to argue that death has occurred when we face the "irreversible" or "permanent" cessation of brain function. Certainly, when blood stops flowing to critical parts of the brain for even a short period of time, the neurons begin to deteriorate and we currently have no way of reversing this damage. "A human life," thought of in terms of brain function (whether higher, lower, or both), "has ended." It is natural, then, to conclude that, although technology has forced us to refine our understanding and has required us to focus on the central biological realities that underlie life and death, the occurrence of death remains an objective event. It is marked by the "irreversible cessation of brain function" and has nothing to do with any decisions we make about it.

But if we pause for a moment, we can see that a key word here, *irreversible*, reflects our current technological limitations.[113] It requires further specification. We cannot now halt or reverse the processes of neuronal deterioration. But we may someday be able to do so. In the future it may be possible, at great cost and effort, to arrest or reverse neuronal death and even to recover substantial brain functioning for some people. If that were so, the span of life, albeit technologically assisted, could extend into the indefinite future. Woody Allen depicts this possibility in his film *Sleeper*. The hero has been cryogenically preserved for centuries (in aluminum foil like a frozen baked potato) and is thawed back to life. Science fiction writers have long imagined such forms of technological resurrection. When this possibility materializes, the value-based choice process already at work in the selection of brain functioning as important to us will become even more evident. The "irreversible cessation of brain function" will be replaced by "what we choose to regard as the irreversible cessation of brain function." When this happens, we will face a number of further questions. Assuming that it will take some time to perfect these techniques, is the possibly diminished functioning we can offer those initially resuscitated worth the opportunity for continued life? How much loss of personality will be tolerable? How will we handle the population problem that results? Are we willing to pay the social costs of preserving and restoring cerebral functioning for thousands or millions of people? Do we really want to postpone "death" in this way? These and other questions will have to be asked and answered. Technology will ensure that death is no longer something "out there," an undeniable biological state that we merely acknowledge. We will have to decide at what point on life's technologically sustainable continuum we will regard someone as unrecoverable and when they will be thought of as "dead" in a moral and legal sense. The choice of biological marker events for declaring life to be at an end will then clearly show itself to be a moral decision.

If limited technological control is one factor obscuring the choice-based nature of our thinking in this area, religion is a second. Historically, life and death, the major boundary points establishing membership in our moral community, have been invested with religious significance. In the biblically based traditions, for example, God is thought of as the governor of life who determines when it starts and ends. In all the traditions that shape our culture, to be alive is to have a living soul, or spirit (Hebrew, *nephesh;* Greek, *pneuma;* Latin, *anima*—all of which are terms originally referring to breath). When the soul, or spirit, departs with our last breath, death ensues. Physically and spiritually, death is "expiration." That the vital principle is described in breath-related terms is not accidental. Spiritual realities are mapped directly onto biological occurrences that once seemed to be definitive marker events. In this way, religion and rudimentary biology worked together to make these events appear as objective, definitive, and independent of any choices on our part. When God is seen as the source of the vital principle, one lives or dies at God's behest. It is not our task to decide these matters, it is God's. We merely understand and acknowledge them.

What was true of our interpretation of life's "end" was also true of its "beginning." Technological limitations, rudimentary understandings of biology, and accompanying religious beliefs together created the appearance of seemingly fixed and meaningful points within continuous biological processes. In the Bible, the first human being, Adam, came into existence at the moment God breathed into the mud of creation. This idea carries over to the individual "creation" events that are believed to mark the start of each subsequent human life. At some moment God acts to form a soul from the pre-existing matrix of matter in the womb, with the result that a unique person comes into being.

Rudimentary biological knowledge supported these ideas. In some traditional societies breath is still regarded as closely associated with the vital principle in human life. Its appearance at birth and departure at death mark the limits of human life.[114] For many centuries Western societies considered the event of "quickening" to be significant. This first manifestation of fetal movement was thought to be the instant when God invests a child with its soul. Early English and American law incorporated this idea by not recognizing harm done to the fetus before quickening. With the advance of medical knowledge, we came to realize that quickening does not represent a real change in the fetus but is only a matter of maternal perception.[115] The search for "objective" events that denote the presence of life in the fetus continued, focusing on earlier events in pregnancy.

This history contributed in the modern period to the investment of fertilization with decisive moral and spiritual significance. Growth in scientific understanding initially fostered this conclusion. The invention of the microscope and the ability to isolate sperm and egg for research purposes allowed us to witness fertilization. What better candidate for the beginning of a human life, when elements from the two parents seem to unite in a single new entity? The later understanding that this union signaled the beginning of major genetic transformations, as chromosomally haploid sex cells became an actively dividing embryo with diploid cells, reinforced the conclusion that this was the decisive "moment" when the human individual began. Older religious ideas of ensoulment contributed to this conclusion. God's intervention to create the spirit was now mapped onto the newly discovered biological information.

But this way of understanding events was bound to be transitory. Newer scientific information has thrown doubt on these certainties. Fertilization, which looked like a "moment," can now be seen as an extended biological process. What seemed like a one-time event—individuation—is now perceived as a process that can continue for up to two weeks. Growth in scientific knowledge has thus highlighted the complexity of these processes and the need for choice in ways that an earlier phase of science, reinforced by ancient religious ideas, helped to obscure.

Against this background, we encounter an important question. If a number of candidate "events" (or points along a continuum) occur that can be selected for the morally important "beginning" or "end" of a human life, how do we determine which we should select? And on what basis do we make the selection? Putting matters in these terms forces our attention away from the events "out there" and draws us reflexively back to the decision process that leads us to identify some occurrence as significant. Our role as active "Copernican" agents comes to the fore.

In thinking about how to select key events in the process of development, it is crucial to understand that boundary markers on the spectrum of human life are important because they govern our bestowal of moral respect. Entities that are deemed to be fully "human" in a moral sense are accorded all the entitlements and protections that go with that status. They are beings whose life cannot ordinarily be taken and who merit all the support we normally give to children and adults. Beings outside this zone have fewer (or no) claims upon us. Humans who cross life's boundary lose these entitlements and protections. We stop our efforts to keep them alive, and, if we have appropriate prior consent, we can harvest their organs for research or transplant purposes.[116] In other words, crucial interests are at stake here. If we place these boundary markers in the wrong place, we risk jeopardizing valuable beings.

We should note that the moral privileges and protections we accord at life's boundary points are not always fully equivalent to those given adult human beings and children. The possibility of relative degrees of respect or protection also exists. For example, although a dead person loses most of the rights of the living, we normally accord the body of the deceased a measure of respect. U.S. law does not accord a fetus the full legal status of a person until birth, but, in the third trimester, the life of a fetus can be taken only to protect the mother's life or health. Thus, moral protection is not always an all-or-nothing matter. Boundary points can be selected to mark increasing (or decreasing) degrees of protection or moral entitlement.

Because boundary markers determine an entity's degree of moral protectedness, why not place them in their most generous locations? Why not push life's moral and legal beginning back to the earliest possible point and thus maximize protections for those embarking on life's journey? Why not push the margin as far out as possible to prevent mistreatment of those departing life? The answer, of course, is that every boundary extension carries a price. These are not cost-free decisions. Every extension of the right to moral protection represents a corresponding burden on those within the moral community who must respect that right. For example, we could expand the perimeter of our thinking about death so that those who are brain dead but whose heart and lungs continue to function with artificial medical support receive full moral protection. Some bioethicists and members of religious groups have supported this expansion because they believe it is offensive to abandon someone who is still breathing and whose heart is beating.[117] But if we accept this conclusion, we may have to sustain indefinitely comatose people on respirators, and we would be prohibited from removing their organs for transplantation. Are we willing to accept this expense and loss? Similarly, at life's beginning, we could push full moral and legal protection back to the earliest possible understanding of fertilization. This would ensure that no tissue that might go on to become a child is intentionally placed at risk. But the price of this in terms of women's freedom alone would be enormous. If, from fertilization onward, the embryo inside a woman's womb were regarded as her moral equivalent, every conflict between the fetus and pregnant woman would require careful determination of whose health and survival should take precedence. If a woman's other interests clashed with the moral claims of the embryo or fetus, those interests could be overridden.

Placing life's moral beginning at this early point would affect not only the pregnant woman and the fetus, but society as a whole. Reproductive embryologists report that human embryos have a very high natural rate of mortality during the first few weeks of development. Estimates vary greatly, but some studies suggest that in normal healthy women, between two-thirds and three-quarters of all fertilized eggs do not go on to implant in the womb.[118] Some of this embryonic loss results from complex biological processes that screen embryos for genetic or chromosomal abnormalities. Embryos that fail to pass this test are sloughed off as a late menstrual period, often without any awareness on the woman's part that she was pregnant. In a sense, early embryonic death is nature's "spell checker." In cases of spontaneous abortion in which a conceptus has been recovered, up to half of the embryos examined have been shown to have chromosomal abnormalities.[119] In view of this high rate of embryonic loss, do we truly want to bestow much moral significance on an entity with which nature is so wasteful? What would be the costs of doing so? If the early embryo is so morally important that we should ban its destruction and forbid research on it that could benefit many children and adults, can we then stand by as thousands or millions of embryos naturally perish each year?[120] Would we not be forced to begin a mammoth medical research program on the order of our "war against cancer" to prevent embryo loss? Committing ourselves to highly value the preimplantation embryo leads to this conclusion.

As the philosopher Mary Anne Warren has observed, if a being has moral status, then "we may not just treat it in any way we please; we are morally obliged to give weight in our deliberations to its needs, interests, or well-being."[121] This means that all our thinking about establishing life's boundaries involves costly choices. What one writer has called the "TANSTAAFL" principle applies: "There Ain't No Such Thing As A Free Lunch."[122] Every expansion of life's boundaries represents a corresponding diminution of living people's rights, liberties, and resources. Determination of a being's status, that is, the selection of appropriate marker events for according moral respect, requires a careful "balancing judgment" in which one must weigh the reasons for selecting any particular point on a developmental path against the reasons for not selecting that point.[123]

This process of selection and decision often involves somewhat arbitrary elements. In matters of moral behavior and law, it is sometimes important that everyone acknowledge the same boundary point as governing their conduct. This can force us to choose some point along a continuum of events. Several candidate points may be available, and we usually end by selecting one for good reasons, although other points could also be chosen. Here, the need to choose is as important as the precise point we select, because, unless we choose a point, things are left unacceptably indeterminate. It is no objection to such choices that the selected point could have been set elsewhere. Nor is it an objection that one is being "inconsistent" in choosing to protect an entity at a certain point when that same entity at a later (or earlier) point possesses many similar qualities. Some point must be chosen along the continuum.[124]

The determination of "majority" provides a good illustration of this. Majority is the age at which an individual attains the full legal rights of adulthood, including the right to vote and the right to make the most important personal decisions. Its determination reveals the complex balancing judgment that occurs in all such boundary choices. On one hand, we want to extend this legal right as far back in age as possible to allow young people greater control over their lives. On the other hand, we know that going back too far might lead to poor decision making that could jeopardize them (in the medical or personal arena) or all of us (in the social and political arenas). So we seek a point of equilibrium between these competing interests. We could select many markers for this purpose: sex-adjusted height or body weight, performance on standardized tests, and so on. All are problematic. In the end, most societies select the arrival at a certain chronological age as the marker event for legal majority. This type of marker is imperfect as well. Not every eighteen-year-old is ready to make important personal or political choices. But we must select some point or risk leaving this crucial area in disarray. A young person at age eighteen is little different than he or she was at age seventeen. Indeed, a youngster who experienced a major life change, perhaps the death of a parent, at age sixteen might be far more mature than most eighteen-year-olds. Nevertheless, we are not being inconsistent in choosing age eighteen, rather than age sixteen or seventeen. Only those who think our choice is driven by some unique and discoverable feature intrinsic to the person will object. These objections fade when we understand that such choices are driven by a complex array of considerations, including such things as the need to choose and the desirability of clear and easily applied markers. In thinking about these important boundary decisions, therefore, we need not be concerned with the charge that our selection is "arbitrary." In this domain, all determinations are "arbitrary" in an etymological sense. They result from willed decisions (Latin *arbitrium* = will). Some choices also involve a deliberate selection of some points over others among a range of good candidates. So long as these choices are made on reasonable grounds, they are not arbitrary in the sense of being merely willful or capricious.

All these considerations ran through my mind as I reviewed the challenge facing our panel with regard to the moral status of the preimplantation embryo. They suggested to me that this issue, like all boundary and status determinations, involves a practical moral choice. Of course, we did not have to decide whether the early embryo is a juridical, legal person meriting equal rights before the law. That had been settled long ago by Anglo-American law, which denies the fetus legal protection until (and unless) it is born. But our panel was being asked to recommend new government regulations for research on the human embryo. The question of the embryo's moral status thus translated into the question of just how much protection it is reasonable and fair to give it at each point in its development. Put another way, how much were we prepared to limit researchers' activities? How much were we willing to put the health of children and adults at risk? At what point is it reasonable to tip the balance in the embryo's favor along the continuum of biological development?

Like all status determinations, answering these questions requires a reasoned, balancing judgment. On one side are considerations prompting us to protect the *ex utero* embryo from mistreatment or death. On the other side are reasons we have for not doing so, including the information and benefits that research might produce. At each point in its development, as the embryo changes, this balancing might also change. Before selecting any specific points as meriting incremental protection, a judgment had to be made about the weight of these reasons in the case before us.

I reviewed in my mind the candidate marker events that were available for according substantial protection to the early embryo. Sperm penetration of the egg was one such marker event. This amounts to locating "fertilization" at this point and forbidding any research beyond it that does not improve the embryo's chances of survival. In favor of this choice is the fact that this event is a reasonably clear point in biological development. Clarity and identifiability are always helpful in choosing boundary markers, because what we are permitting or prohibiting should be readily understandable by everyone affected by our decision (one of the reasons chronological age is so appealing for the choice of the age of majority).

The events surrounding sperm penetration, particularly the locking out of other sperm, also represent a great increase in an entity's potential for development into a human being. Whether an entity's potential for development to adult human status should be among our reasons for protecting it is one of the most disputed questions in the philosophical literature.[125] Many natural entities have the potential for further development, but they nevertheless lack the value they attain in their mature state. Eggs cost less than chickens; acorns are not oaks.[126] Even so, a greatly increased likelihood that an entity will go on to become an identifiable human being has some significance. Emotionally and conceptually, we hesitate to permit the destruction of something that seems to be clearly on its way to being "one of us." Along the continuum of subtle transformations, increased potential for development at sperm penetration thus represents a relatively distinct biological occurrence that might make this point an attractive marker event for the beginning of a being's right to moral respect.

Nevertheless, a number of considerations militate against selecting this point as decisive. Sperm often penetrate eggs that then cease to develop. This renders the potentiality argument somewhat less compelling. Setting the boundary here would also foreclose research aimed at learning about complex processes of sperm penetration and cytoplasmic activation in the egg. This research often requires the destruction of the fertilized ovum. The information derived from this research is very important for the development of new contraceptives and for understanding the causes of many common birth defects resulting from polyspermic fertilization. In light of the important potential benefits of such research, legislators in Victoria, Australia, chose syngamy rather than sperm penetration as the crucial marker event. Legislation there prohibits research that destroys the embryo but permits it "from the point of sperm penetration prior to but not including the point of syngamy."[127] Is this choice arbitrary? It is certainly not obvious that a new kind of being starts when the zygote's two sets of chromosomes line up next to each other rather than being separated by several thousandths of a millimeter of egg cytoplasm. But the Australian legislators apparently decided they did not want to forgo all the benefits of reproductive research. Is this a good choice? Should the cut-off point be located even later in the course of development? If so, how much later? To answer these questions, we can move onward and look carefully at the array of benefits and harms associated with the next available marker event, syngamy.

Choosing to cut off all nontherapeutic manipulations of the embryo at syngamy has some clear benefits. Now we have an entity that looks and acts even more like a diploid cell, even though it still lacks a nuclear membrane and its paternal set of chromosomes remains inactive for days. Syngamy, too, is a marker event that satisfies the requirements of clarity and identifiability of boundaries. If there were no other considerations, this might be a good point to establish considerable moral protection and impose strict limitations on research that leads to the destruction of the embryo.

But some important considerations exist on the other side of the issue. Granting a high degree of moral status to the embryo at this point—and correspondingly prohibiting all research that leads to its destruction—means that we lose many of the benefits that people like Jonathan Van Blerkom, Maria Bustillo, and others told us that research can bring. By continuing to study the embryo beyond syngamy through its earliest cleavage stages and by permitting interventions that are incompatible with its further development, we can very likely develop safer and more efficient infertility procedures, more effective contraceptives, and better ways of understanding and preventing birth defects and pediatric cancers. If we foreclose this kind of research on the developing preimplantation embryo, in other words, living women and children face a greater risk of death or disease than is necessary. This is not speculation. The high morbidity and mortality associated with the epidemic of high-order multiple births is the most glaring consequence of poorly researched infertility procedures. In the words of Axel Kahn, a member of France's national bioethics committee, assisted reproduction is the only field of medicine in which the success or failure of experiments is established by the state of a born child.[128]

Understanding what is at stake here forces us to look even more closely at this crucial choice. Given the costs, why would we want to select a point so early as syngamy? Some might reply by referring to my observations about biological occurrences as processes rather than events. We should choose this early marker, they might say, precisely because there are no clear events beyond it on the continuum of embryonic development. Once the line is crossed that leads to a self-developing embryo, change is continuous. We have seen that clear markers are valuable when conduct affecting basic rights and entitlements is involved. Unless the protective boundaries constitute bright lines, research that harms the early embryo could lead to the abuse of older research subjects, including more developed fetuses, newborns, or even children. This way of thinking draws on a "slippery slope" argument. It is a reasonable source of worry. In establishing moral boundaries, we should always try to achieve confidence that our lines are clear and sustainable.[129] But the concern here to avail ourselves of the clear lines that sperm penetration or syngamy represent rests on the assumption that other, later marker events cannot be found that would permit us to impose sustainable restrictions. For example, we could instead select the appearance of the primitive streak as the decisive marker event. This point, too, is relatively clear and identifiable. It is easily observable under the microscope and, as we identify the gene products that induce it, it may someday be subject to a simple genetic assay. It signals the end of the possibility of twinning and recombination. It encompasses a period during which some of the most basic events of embryogenesis occur and when the embryo is particularly susceptible to developmental failures caused by genetic problems or toxins in the maternal environment. It also currently represents the far limit of our ability to sustain a human embryo *in vitro* for research purposes. At the present time, human embryos cannot be kept alive *in vitro* for more than a few days. It will be years before techniques are available that allow them to develop normally in the laboratory up to the point of gastrulation.

There are other good reasons for selecting the appearance of the primitive streak as an end point for research that risks harm to the embryo. Within days of this, neuralation, the earliest formation of the nervous system, begins. The neural tube then progresses to the essential subdivisions of the brain into forebrain, midbrain, and hindbrain.[130] It is very unlikely that sentience, the capacity to feel pleasure or pain, starts at this point. For that, much greater development of the nervous system, weeks or months later, is needed.[131] Nevertheless, sentience cannot be ruled out absolutely after this point, as it can before any nervous system tissue is present. The very high natural rate of mortality during the first two weeks of development is also a relevant consideration here. As I have said, it would be odd to accord early embryos a high degree of moral protection when so many of them are routinely lost through normal biological processes.

I have said nothing about the embryo's own stake in these matters. Almost all moral theories require us to consider the impact of our choices and acts on all those whom they might affect.[132] For example, if we choose to set legal majority at age 21, we have to consider how we would feel about this if we were younger people who might thereby be denied the vote. If we choose the irreversible cessation of total brain function as the defining point of death, we have to ask ourselves whether we would be willing to have medical treatments stopped for us when our brain had ceased functioning in this way. Of course, taking others' interests and points of view into account does not mean that we have to end by protecting or privileging those interests. The widespread acceptance of brain death indicates that, apart from respectful treatment of our remains, most of us do not care about what happens to us once our brain has stopped functioning. Our interest in maintaining ourselves when only our heart and lungs are functioning is minimal.

It follows that we must also consider the impact of our choices on the tiny, multicellular organism that is the early embryo. How would we feel if, as an embryo, we were subjected to research manipulations that led to our death? Even as I state this question, however, we can see how odd it is. How do we think about our concerns or "interests" as a very early human embryo? On the basis of everything we know about biology, it seems reasonable to say that the preimplantation embryo itself has no thoughts or feelings. As a collection of undifferentiated cells, it possesses no tissues and none of the nervous system structures needed for mental activities. If I were an embryo I certainly would have no feelings. Yet each one of us was, at one time, an embryo. Would we have wanted then to be regarded as a research subject who could be manipulated and destroyed?

Of course, none of us would want to be harmed as an embryo when it was likely that we would be transferred back to a womb for eventual birth. If I were injured as an embryo and then returned to my mother's womb, I might have been born as a severely damaged child who could have grown into an impaired adult. Permitting such activities risks all of our lives and health. But the object of harm here is the born child and the adult it becomes. None of us wants to permit practices that lead to living children and adults being injured. This means that research performed on early embryos intended for transfer back to a womb should either be harmless or aim at improving the survival and health of the resulting child.

If this standard is adopted, we should not permit research on an embryo that could lead to harm for a born child produced from it. This means either that no such research will be done, or that researchers will take care not to transfer back to a womb any embryo on which such research has been done. What are we to say, then, about my interests and feelings as an embryo that, by the very nature of the research protocol, will not be transferred and is destined never to be born?

In asking this question, we enter a domain where reasoning follows unfamiliar paths and where linguistic mirages confront us at every turn. Take, for example, the question "Would I be willing to allow embryos to be used in research and then discarded?" It is easy to convert this into the question "Would I be willing to be used in harmful research without my consent and then killed or allowed to die?" However, these are two different questions. The embryo is not yet a conscious adult who can anticipate or experience its own death. We are not talking about the killing of an adult or pediatric research subject. Instead, what is involved here is a decision to halt the development of an entity that might go on to become a sentient being and, then, a conscious human being. A more appropriate way of putting the question is "Would I want to be used without my consent in research that leads to my never developing beyond the status of an early embryo?"

This question is closer to the right one, but it, too, can be linguistically misleading. A condition of asking it is that I am already here. No one who asks this question will *ever* face the prospect of never having been allowed to develop into a person. However, because our language permits us to ask this question from the point of view of a living person with a clear interest in his or her life, it easily, but erroneously, slips over into a very different question: "Would I as a living person want the life that I have lived to vanish from the world as though I had never been?" Hardly anyone wants to disappear in this way. But this, too, is a very different matter from never having developed beyond the status of an early embryo—from never having become an identifiable, conscious individual in the first place.

Avoiding these linguistic illusions, we reach what seems to be a clearer way of putting the question: "Is 'someone' harmed when, once conceived, they do not progress beyond the stage of an early embryo?" When stated in this way, the question, though still perplexing and unfamiliar, is more amenable to being answered. One thing we can do is draw on the moral common sense of other human beings. How do most people actually feel about the very early embryo? How much concern do they evidence when an embryo fails to implant or grow and develop beyond very early pregnancy? In reply to this question, it does not seem to strike most of us as a significant source of concern when early embryos fail to develop. This is reflected in the willingness of those couples who desperately want a baby to produce many more embryos in infertility procedures than they plan to use. One study of such couples in Belgium found that ninety-two percent of those who freeze embryos in connection with their infertility treatments approved of the eventual destruction of surplus embryos. Although fifty-nine percent of these couples identified themselves as Roman Catholic, no difference in the willingness to destroy surplus embryos was found with regard to religion.[133]

This same indifference to the fate of early embryos is reflected in our relative unconcern about very early miscarriages, those in the first few weeks of a pregnancy. Although miscarriages can be deeply upsetting events when they occur after a pregnancy is well established, they can also be troubling even in the first weeks of a pregnancy when they signal a difficulty to conceive. The emotional weight here usually stems from the problems they indicate in one's ability to have a child. But very early miscarriages are not usually mourned as deeply as later miscarriages. A similar indifference to the loss of early embryos is reflected in the nearly universal neglect of the fact that the large majority of embryos never actually implant in the womb. Medical specialists have known about this high rate of early embryo loss for years, but no one has ever lamented it as one of the great tragedies facing humanity. No one has proposed a "National Institute for the Prevention of Early Embryo Mortality." No "pro-life" spokesperson has ever denounced this medical neglect of a whole class of human beings. Behind these attitudes lies a sense that the very beginnings of life are too precarious and too lacking in the qualities we care about (like feeling and consciousness) to elicit much concern on our part. Just as we do not much care about the treatment of those who are brain dead, we do not seem to care about the fate of the many rudimentary human entities that naturally never get beyond the embryonic stage.

These considerations suggest that the early embryo's interests are not among those we need take into account in establishing boundary points to protect it. Because it is not sentient, it is not physically harmed by its use in research, and its loss of opportunity to come into being is not something we appear to regard as a significant concern. Very bluntly (and excusing the use of unavoidably misleading language), one can say "I would not have cared if I had been discarded as an embryo."[134]

The objection can be made that these attitudes are morally unsound. The philosopher Don Marquis, for example, has affirmed in a widely reprinted article that killing is immoral because it is wrong, except in extreme circumstances, to cause "the loss to the victim of the value of the victim's future."[135] It is this deprivation, and not the specific acts of violence or the harms associated with most killing, that is objectionable. Certainly Marquis is right concerning living humans. We have a great deal of emotional investment in our future, and to be deprived of it against our will, however painlessly, is a great wrong.[136] But does this logic apply to the early conceptus that has never lived and is incapable of anticipating a future? I think not. Our almost universal indifference to the natural deaths of the great majority of conceptuses supports this conclusion.[137]

A further objection is worth considering. Someone might say, "Of course you do not mind the neglect of embryos, but this is only because you are among those already *here*. Your thinking reflects the fact that you have survived to adulthood. What about all those others who are not so lucky? Are you not being too much influenced by the fact that you know you have made it to life outside the womb? Yours is not really a moral attitude, but a self-centered way of thinking."

The force of this objection derives from an important requirement of moral reasoning. We must always consider not only the impact of conduct on ourselves but also its implications for all as a generally permitted rule of conduct.[138] Many forms of conduct exist that can never possibly threaten me because of the particular situation I have reached in life. Consider the issue of whether we should tolerate child abuse. I will never again be a child. If I permit abuse to happen, I know that I will not be directly victimized. Nevertheless, if I am to reason morally, I must not only put myself in others' shoes but also consider the impact of the behavior I propose as a generally approved mode of conduct. As an allowable practice, child abuse would affect many people into the indefinite future. If it were something generally permitted in society, it might even have affected me, and I would be suffering today as a result. In assessing conduct, I must always look to these abiding implications of a permitted form of conduct for all members of society.

But this requirement need not alter our thinking about not sustaining very early embryos. Where this conduct is permitted, there never will be a conscious child or adult human being who will suffer or who will have reason to regret the practice. In other words, the treatment of very early embryos represents an odd case in which our "partiality" in favoring born and conscious beings is morally acceptable. The failure to sustain the embryos is a form of conduct which, by its very nature, will never be experienced as a harm by "anyone" who could care. Only a moral "optical illusion" involving the over-imaginative application of impartiality leads us to think that, in this case, we are being "unfair" by not considering the interests of an entity we can never be.

One final objection is worth considering. Someone may say that dismissing as unimportant the embryo's stake in coming into being misrepresents what an embryo is. "There is no question of the embryo's not coming into being. It already is in being. The embryo is not like sex cells in the parents' bodies that may or may not join to produce a new life. Once fertilization occurs, something decisive has happened. From this point on, a being exists who, regardless of what it may experience, intrinsically merits respect and whose development should not be stopped arbitrarily."

This is the prevalent way of thinking. Many people believe that fertilization (however defined) is a decisive marker event and that the embryo, because it becomes a human being at this time, has important moral claims. But this objection wholly misses the point I have been making. Instead of starting with the need to argue for the merit of selecting boundary points on life's continuum, it begins with the certainty that something morally significant happens at fertilization and that this "something" merits moral respect. I have been arguing just the opposite. There are no self-evident boundary lines "out there." Many points can qualify as morally significant in the complex sequence of events that marks biological development. The choice of one over another is not obvious and must be backed up by good reasons that take into account both the benefits and harms of that choice for us all. Some of those who "see" fertilization as morally decisive do so by invoking particular religious beliefs not shared by others. Others exercise their reason and make the complex decision that around this time in the reproductive process enough change has happened to recommend a high degree of moral respect for the developing embryo. Both viewpoints may be correct. Perhaps this is a spiritually significant point; perhaps this is a good place to commence substantial moral protection. But if so, it is a choice that must be justified through argument. One cannot merely assert that at this point the embryo is morally different from anything else on the biological spectrum. It must be shown clearly what the difference is and why it is important enough for us to severely limit our liberty with respect to it, including our liberty of health-related research. In making this argument we must follow the pattern of reasoning I have traced. We must identify the benefits and harms associated with the choice of a particular boundary point, including the benefits and harms to the entity under consideration. On this basis, we must indicate why it is reasonable to select any point as meriting an enhanced degree of moral protection.

Over the years, I have made these arguments in many writings and lectures. In doing so, I learned that even to suggest that these matters involve choices and decisions on our part invites this response: "No choice is involved here. This moment (fertilization or whatever) clearly marks the start of moral status." Why is this view so prevalent? Why do people typically insist that we merely identify life's boundary markers and vehemently deny that we choose them? I think there are at least several reasons. One is the continuing influence of religion. Beneath the surface reality of biological occurrences, many of us still see decisive spiritual events. Looking at the embryo, watching its miraculous progress from sperm penetration through early development, it is easy for those raised in a religious environment to see God's hand.[139] Because moral agents usually make meaningful choices when they act, and because choice usually occurs in a seemingly "timeless" instant of resolve, it is natural to think that God, the supreme moral agent, acts similarly when He intervenes spiritually to start a new life. If we begin with the assumption that God is active in human conception and birth, it is natural to perceive decisive and meaningful events amidst the continua that mark biological development. What better candidate for a decisive event than fertilization, the moment when multiplicity seems to become singularity and dramatically new developmental energies are unleashed?

All of this may be true. Sperm penetration, syngamy, or some other candidate for the "moment of fertilization" may, in fact, be spiritually significant. No one can say that this is untrue. But religious views such as these cannot be the basis for public policy in a pluralistic, religiously diverse society. If the matter were cost-free, we might choose to respect religious positions on these matters. Because we must choose some line, why not choose one that happens to fit some major religious groups' spiritual understanding of life's beginning? But if we accept an early cut-off point for the permissibility of research, little doubt exists that the health of women involved in infertility procedures and the children produced by these procedures will be adversely affected. Many people will be deprived of the benefits of new scientific and medical information. Why should some people's religiously shaped views and preferences override these pressing health concerns? Public policy formation in this area, therefore, demands that all arguments for and against particular boundary points be subjected to critical scrutiny. Religiously based views cannot be exempted from this requirement.

Remarkably, it is not only religiously minded people who approach these questions searching for objective conditions to determine judgment. The conviction that establishing life's moral boundaries involves no choices but merely the identification of objective states, or properties "out there" in the biological organism, continues to play a powerful role, even among secular thinkers and philosophers. In the abortion controversy, for example, this conviction contributes to a tendency for people to alight on one or another property of the entity, usually something intrinsic to it, that is presented as definitive of "humanness" or "personhood." This way of thinking is another reason why people tend to miss the role of choice in our determination of boundary markers.

Examples of this habit of mind are found on both sides of the abortion debate. On the conservative side, we find people arguing that humanness is the existence (at fertilization and beyond) of a unique genetic identity: "A being who possesses all the genetic features of a human being is a human being."[140] In this kind of stipulative, definitional approach, there is usually no hint of the presence of a complex moral argument involving reasoned choice. More fully developed, the argument could involve the claim that, all things considered, the formation of a new genetic identity is the best boundary marker we can select for establishing full moral protection. But to open the argument fully in this way would expose it to critical analysis. Is it really true that the emergence of a new genetic identity is the best boundary marker we can select? The tendency to avoid this question and the effort to approach the matter definitionally ("humanness = "possessing a diploid genome") reflect a closed-minded strategy aimed at avoiding reasoned argument. That this strategy can succeed—or even seem to be reasonable—shows how deeply rooted is our tendency to reduce these matters to the identification of objective events or properties in the organism.

The conservative side of the abortion debate is not alone in approaching the problem in this way. On the pro-choice side, a series of competing biological or psychological properties have frequently been offered as definitionally constitutive of personhood. Sentience,[141] brain activity,[142] and self-concept or self-awareness[143] have all been said to be definitive of what it means for something to be deserving of moral protection and "human" in a moral sense. These definitional proposals possess the argumentative advantage of denying the early fetus significant moral protection and grounding a woman's right of access to abortion, but they lead to a series of moral perplexities. For example, stress on sentience as a reason for substantial moral protection brings many animals into the same zone of moral protection as well-developed human fetuses. This might preclude the use of animals for food or medical experimentation, a conclusion that only a few die-hard animal rights advocates wish to defend.[144] Stress on self-awareness or self-concept can also have the effect of excluding most newborn and very young children from the zone of protection. Faced with these perplexities, some who hold these positions have been forced to accept the intuitively offensive implications of their definition, including the view that infanticide is morally permissible,[145] or have tried to jerry-rig solutions to the problem the definition creates. One defender of the self-concept definition, for example, argues that although newborns are not definitionally human in a moral sense, our respect for parents' feelings counsels a rigorous ban on infanticide.[146]

All these problems stem from the failure to realize that the judgments of "humanity," "personhood," or any similar determination of moral protectedness are not a matter of definition, of finding the intrinsic biological property of an entity that makes it morally protectable, but are instead the outcome of a complex moral choice involving many competing considerations. Sometimes these considerations have less to do with the nature of the entity than with the implications of a boundary marker itself. For example, birth is an excellent boundary marker for establishing full and equal moral protection for human beings. It is a definitive event, easily recognized. It represents a point at which the physical claims to life of mother and child can no longer conflict. It brings the child into the world, where its mistreatment can profoundly implicate others, not just its parents. It marks the beginning of a continuous process of development, beyond which few firm boundary markers exist (if we permit the killing of one-day-olds, why not one-month-olds, and so on?). Yet, except for the fact that the infant before birth is still attached to the placenta and the newborn can breathe on its own, the child just before birth and the newborn are biologically almost identical. To try to understand the choice of birth in terms of biological features of the child can thus lead to serious moral confusion. For example, we might try to understand this boundary in terms of some intrinsic property of the child that is "necessary and sufficient" for full moral entitlement, a property that the child attains only at birth. One prospect here is a child's "ability to breathe on its own." But if we follow this route, we may be forced to exclude from the moral community premature newborns who are sustained on ventilators, even though, in terms of most of the features that make birth a good marker, these infants qualify: they are out of their mother's womb, they are independent individuals in our midst, we medically neglect them at our moral peril, and so on.[147] The mistake here is to take one feature of a complex boundary marker choice—in this case, the fact that most babies who have been born happen to breathe on their own—and make this the defining feature behind that choice, when, in fact, the choice results from a variety of considerations, no one of which is decisive.

Against this background, we can see why efforts to define humanity in terms of a single intrinsic property, such as genetic identity, rationality, or self-awareness, go awry. All these efforts begin by focusing on some feature normally present in beings that we acknowledge as deserving of moral protection. Working on the assumption that determining humanity in a moral sense is a matter of identifying that property, they then make this feature a necessary and sufficient condition for the possession of full moral protectedness. But this approach misses the fact that protectedness is established by the choice of a marker event for which a variety of independent, intersecting, and compelling reasons exist, some of which have little to do with the properties of the entity itself. It is true that we normally value our lives because we are self-conscious and rational, but we extend protection to others who lack these qualities when there are good reasons for doing so. Newborns are not rational and are only minimally self-conscious, but we choose to include them in our moral community, regardless of their cognitive status, for many good reasons. These include the fact that most of us tend to intensely love our young and that we are aware that neglect or abuse of children can have catastrophic consequences for all.[148]

Inclusion of newborns in our moral community is often pointed to by those who prefer to choose sentience, rather than rationality or self-consciousness, as a decisive qualifying property for moral protection. However, they, too, miss the complexity of these choices. Sentience is certainly one consideration in boundary-drawing activities, but it cannot be taken as definitive without attention to all the implications of doing so. For example, it is very common for those who stress sentience as the chief qualifying ground for an entity's meriting protection to brand as "speciesist" anyone who denies animals the same degree of moral protection we accord human infants.[149] If infants, who lack higher cognitive abilities, are protected because they are sentient, how can we rationally exclude animals, whose abilities to suffer pain are equivalent? But this argument misses the point that these protection decisions are not based on the identification of a single, defining property in the entity. They result from a variety of complex considerations, including those having to do with human survival and well being. We feel special obligations to protect our young for all the reasons I have mentioned. The treatment of animals and their inclusion in our zone of protection poses an altogether different set of questions. Some animals threaten our lives, and we must be prepared to kill them to protect our own lives. Others are useful sources of food or clothing and would not even exist in large numbers if we did not domesticate them. This does not mean that we can neglect the importance of sentience as a consideration inducing us to extend some degree of moral protection. This is one basis for our animal protection laws, as well as many people's objections to cruel "factory farming" methods of food production. Nevertheless, it is mistaken to make sentience the necessary and sufficient basis of an entity's claim to moral protectability. It is *one* consideration to which others must be added. Only those who see matters of moral protectedness as involving the identification of some key property in a class of beings and who fail to see the total process of reasoned choice involved will view as rationally inconsistent our conduct in placing sentient animals outside the zone of full and equal protection where our newborn children reside.[150] That all these views that start with some defining feature of what makes a being protectable are so prevalent in abortion debates testifies to the enduring hold of the idea that we must look for some intrinsic property "out there" in the entity the possession of which compels us to grant the entity moral protection.

A final reason for resistance to the idea that these boundary matters proceed from reasoned choices also leads back, albeit indirectly, to the role of religion in shaping our thinking. Many people fear that acknowledging the role of human reason and decision in such vital matters will imperil whole classes of vulnerable human beings. Those who express this fear sometimes point to the tendency of human beings to dehumanize their foes. The Nazis' branding of Jews, Slavs, and others as racially and biologically "subhuman" illustrates what can happen when basic matters of human rights are made subject to some group's decision.[151] In view of these recognized perils, is it not safer to identify objective features of development, such as fertilization, that cast the net of moral protectedness as wide as possible and minimize the risk of arbitrary exclusion? Some further argue that it is an error to see these matters in terms of human choice at all. Instead, we should rely on religious authority and tradition for guidance. Only this transcendent foundation guarantees that no single human group will ever be in a position to mistreat others. Many who hold this view also typically perceive fertilization as a divinely established boundary marker.

These objections and fears are understandable, but they fundamentally misrepresent the issues. For one thing, it is a parody of the need for reasoned choice in these matters to equate it to the terrible instances of racial exclusion and genocide that have occurred in the past. Boundary decisions about life's beginning and end affect us all and must be thought of as being made by us all. No one capable of engaging in reasoned discussion can arbitrarily be excluded from participating in making them. They must also be made with the maximal degree of objectivity and impartiality we can achieve, and they must embrace the interests of everyone affected by them. In this respect, they are no different than any other decisions we make about human rights. Just as it is wrong to exclude whole groups of citizens from the right to vote because of their race or ethnicity, so arbitrary and unjustified exclusions have no place in the boundary determining process for human community and moral protections.

The preference for "objective" markers identified through biology or religion also obscures the fact that *any* selection of a boundary marker is a choice. Those who point to fertilization as the safest criterion as a marker for full moral protection are making a choice. Their reasons for doing so may be rational or religious, but they are reasons that must be brought to the surface. There is no alternative to human choice in this arena (even the choice of a religious solution). The only alternative to self-conscious choice prepared to openly defend its assumptions and conclusions is hidden choice that obscures its decisional basis. Once we see that human choice underlies all these matters, we also perceive that the problem of arbitrary abuse and exclusion is not confined to a view that is open about its decisional basis and choice criteria. Exclusion and abuse can occur whenever human beings seek moral advantage by means of boundary determinations. Just as the Nazi experience illustrates the presence of prejudice and the gross misuse of science to defend unjustified exclusions, many conservative religious positions on abortion display serious neglect of women's interests in reaching their conclusions. The alternative to abuse and exclusion is not to obscure the need for choice and decision in these matters, but to make choice explicit and to be prepared rationally to defend one's criteria before the entire human moral community. Every member of this community has a vital stake in these matters, and every person has a right to be aware of and to participate in these determinations. Taking concrete steps toward realizing this ideal of inclusiveness and transparency in our debates about the boundaries of moral protection is the best way to prevent unjust exclusion and scapegoating.

Reviewing all these matters in my mind, I knew they would deeply influence my approach to preparing a draft section on the embryo's moral status. But I also realized that a public document like this was no place to develop every feature of this thought process. The challenge, therefore, was to move from this complex structure to a series of brief, clear, and compelling arguments grounding the practical conclusions to which they led. As an ethicist, I strongly believed that a principled argument was necessary in any report prepared by the panel. A decade earlier, the Warnock Committee approached a similar challenge and produced a document that largely bypassed moral reasoning. Dame Warnock and her colleagues opted merely to state the feelings of most members of the committee about the matters under review. In many instances, the only explanation for positions taken is the statement "a majority of the committee believes. . . ."[152] The Canadian Royal Commission on Reproductive Technology took a similar approach in its lengthy two-volume report issued just the year before our panel was convened.[153] Drawing on an extensive process of gathering the views of many Canadians through various public meetings, the commission's report repeatedly used the phrase "the majority of Canadians believes . . ." to justify its recommendations. It would be unfair to say that either the Warnock or Canadian report is devoid of moral reasoning, but what is striking about both documents is the lack of substantial reasoned arguments for their positions. However difficult it might be, I told myself, our panel's report would avoid these vague appeals to majority sentiment and would try to offer a reasoned defense of our recommendations. As the philosopher Dan Brock noted, the ability of a public ethics commission to settle moral disputes rests not on how its members vote but on the quality of the arguments it offers.[154]

In the brief period before the 14 March meeting, Carol Tauer and I communicated extensively by e-mail and phone. We agreed that I would write a statement about the moral status of the early embryo and that Carol would focus on whether, if we permitted some forms of embryo research, we should impose a time limit on how long an embryo could be allowed to develop before research on it had to stop. Both of us would jointly begin to put together some reflections on the difficult issue of whether it is ever permissible to fertilize eggs only for research purposes when there is no intention of returning the resulting embryo to a womb for development and birth. This is different from the use of embryos left over from infertility procedures that were going to be destroyed in any case. Carol had thought about this issue more than I had. To catch up, I decided to consult extensively with Brigid Hogan, our science co-chair, about why this possibility might be scientifically or medically important. Carol and I hoped to bring together these various issues in a brief document, between ten and fifteen pages long, to submit to Pat King as one part of the policy discussions of our planned report.

As the March meeting neared, something happened that had a powerful impact on my thinking. I received a call from someone who introduced himself as a radiation oncologist at the Norris Cotton Cancer Center at the Dartmouth-Hitchcock Medical Center. "I understand that you're serving on the NIH embryo panel," he said. "Would you be willing to meet with me? I have some things that I'd like to talk over with you." I replied that I would be glad to do so. We arranged to have lunch together.

Entering his office a few days later, I was surprised to see a man in his early forties confined to a wheelchair. Over lunch he explained to me that he had been injured a few years before when his plane crashed during a snowstorm at Denver's Stapleton Airport. Others had died, and he was lucky to survive, but he was now paralyzed from the waist down. Looking at me across the luncheon table, he said, "I wanted to meet with you to tell you that the work your panel is doing is very important. Embryo research is crucial to me—personally and professionally. For one thing, assisted reproductive technologies are the only way I can have my own children. For another, research on the early development of nervous system tissue is a major source of hope for me, and those like me, who have suffered spinal cord injuries."

He went on to explain that most nervous system tissue does not grow or repair itself after the stages of early embryonic and fetal development. The reasons for this failure are poorly understood, but one consequence is that nerve damage caused by trauma or disease is usually permanent. If it were possible to return adult neurons to their pluripotent embryonic stage and stimulate them to resume growth, paraplegics like him could recover their mobility. Individuals who have suffered damage to the optic or auditory nerves could recover sight or hearing. The ancient dream of the lame walking and the blind seeing might become reality.

What this colleague was saying was not entirely new to me. During our first panel meeting, science co-chair Brigid Hogan had mentioned the possibility of developing pluripotent embryonic stem cells lines as a way of providing tissue for transplant purposes in the treatment of blood, nervous system, and other disorders. But now Brigid's mention of promising research directions had a human face. Here was a bright, young physician whose life had been marred by a tragic accident and who, like many others, might be assisted by the applications resulting from embryo research. In the weeks and months ahead, this conversation with my colleague never left my mind. As I turned to the task of determining how we should treat the tiny, multicellular embryo, I realized that whatever claims it might have would have to be weighed against the urgent health needs of thousands of people like him.

3

DRAFTING A REPORT

═══════════════════════════

THE panel's three days of meetings in March and April were enormously productive. They gave us a chance to gather and critique the work of smaller subgroups. In the course of these meetings, broad areas of consensus on ethical and policy issues emerged. Naturally, questions remained to be discussed or voted on, and islands of prose had to be bridged by our newly appointed science writer, Kathi Hanna. But from late April onward we could see the outlines of a final report.

Much of this progress was the result of hard work by science co-chair Brigid Hogan. Brigid's personality shaped the panel's work from the start. Raised in Britain in strapped economic circumstances by a widowed mother, Brigid had gone on to a distinguished university career and an appointment to the Medical Research Council, Britain's counterpart of the NIH. Her work there led to the offer of a professorship at Vanderbilt University, where she headed a laboratory working on mouse embryology and genetics. Everything in Brigid's past convinced her of the value of scientific research. For her, engaging in poor-quality science was a cardinal sin, and willed ignorance about anything that good research could shed light on was unthinkable.

Like John Eppig and others who worked with mice, Brigid was aware that the preceding decade had seen great strides in understanding embryo development in other mammals but that little of this work had yet been applied to human beings. After consulting with several other leading scientists on the panel and elsewhere, Brigid put together a draft of what would eventually become the first chapter of our report. It was an overview of the types of potentially valuable research that might be undertaken with NIH support—a kind of scientific "wish list" of research possibilities. In it, Brigid avoided making moral judgments while offering clear explanations in lay terms of the more complex research areas.

The 14 March meeting began with Brigid making a brief oral presentation of key points in her draft document. Near the top of the list in terms of immediate usefulness, she emphasized, was research aimed at improving the safety and efficiency of assisted reproductive procedures. Although thousands of women each year are routinely administered Pergonal or Clomid to stimulate them to produce enough eggs for fertilization, little is known about the effects of these powerful drugs. In an estimated one-in-fifty *in vitro* fertilization (IVF) cycles, high-dose ovarian stimulation leads to what is known as "severe ovarian hyperstimulation syndrome."[155] This condition involves dramatic enlargement of the ovaries and life-threatening fluid imbalances. It is also possible that these infertility drugs may damage immature eggs in women's ovaries and be one cause of the relatively high rate of failure to implant of eggs produced in IVF procedures. Some studies had suggested, but not proven, a possible link between these drugs and ovarian cancer.[156] Research could shed light on these matters and, in the short run, lead to lower dosages in current stimulation regimens.

Brigid's own research interests evidenced themselves in other items on the list. Embryonic development is the most biologically active period in an organism's life. At each moment, rapidly dividing cells emit and receive chemical signals to produce the gene products that are the body's building blocks. Embryo research might allow us to identify these signals and create immortalized biochemical "libraries" of expressed genes (cDNA's). Correlated with embryonic development, these cDNA libraries could help us understand the functional roles of thousands of genes. This could lead to new drug therapies for health problems in children or adults caused when gene expression breaks down or goes awry later in life.

Brigid's draft chapter and her presentation wound up with a discussion of the possibility of using human embryos to develop pluripotent stem cell lines. These cell lines had already been developed in the mouse, she explained. Brigid had actually pioneered some of the relevant techniques.[157] An embryo that was not transferred to a womb at an early date could not continue normal development *in vitro* because it lacked the support structures of the womb. However, if culturing were continued *in vitro* with proper growth factors, an embryo would form a layer of unspecialized or semispecialized stem cells able to produce an abundance of blood, nervous system, bone, skin, or other tissues. These could be further cultured to make immortal cell lines that, because of their prolificness and ability to permit selection from among a range of types for the lowest possible immune reaction, could have a host of medical applications in people whose own tissues had broken down. As Brigid spoke, it occurred to me that the realization of my injured Dartmouth colleague's dream of nervous system repair started here.

Mark Hughes of the Baylor College of Medicine followed Brigid with a slide presentation of his work in the area of preimplantation genetic diagnosis (PGD). Mark's presence on the panel eventually became a major source of controversy, fueling the charge that the panel as a whole was composed of scientists seeking funding for their own work. These charges reached a crescendo when, in June, Mark accepted an appointment to continue his research on PGD at the NIH's Center for Human Genome Research. Mark's research opportunities in this post would be greatly enhanced if we recommended federal funding for embryo research. But when Mark was appointed to the panel, he had no idea that he would eventually be offered a position at the NIH. No doubt the appearance of conflict created by Mark's multiple involvements spawned criticisms of our work. Nevertheless, I believe these criticisms were unfair. Mark was a researcher at the very forefront of one of the most important areas within our purview. Presumably, he was asked to serve because of his understanding of the scientific issues in this area. Not to have Mark on the panel would have represented a major loss of expertise. These conflicts are built into the NIH peer-review process, which relies on leading people in a field to determine the direction of future funding. Avoiding conflict of interest altogether in these areas would leave the direction of research either to government science administrators or to scientists whose own work was so poor that they could not qualify for federal support.

Mark's presentation reviewed the limited options open to couples who wish to have a child but who know that they carry genes likely to cause a serious genetic disorder. They can pursue adoption, or they can seek to establish a pregnancy with donor gametes. If neither of these choices is acceptable to them—as is true for many people—the current alternative is to start a pregnancy and then undergo chorionic villus sampling (CVS) at ten to twelve weeks gestation age or amniocentesis at sixteen weeks. In either case, if genetic testing shows the fetus to be affected, the couple faces the prospect of terminating a well-established pregnancy. Mark reported that he had initially believed that PGD would be most attractive to people who were morally opposed to abortion, but he was surprised to learn that only about thirty percent of people using the new technology reported doing so for this reason. The majority of couples may already have had one abortion to prevent the birth of an affected child, he told us, and they sought PGD because late-term abortions are "a family nightmare."[158] PGD allows couples instead to undergo an IVF procedure followed by a molecular analysis of the resulting embryos. Only those embryos found to be free of the disease (or who are merely carriers of a recessive disorder) are transferred. Because couples in whom one or both partners carry a problematic gene usually are not also having infertility problems, establishing a pregnancy is much easier when PGD is used than with most IVF procedures.

Mark's presentation ended with a slide of a child born to a family who had recently undergone a PGD procedure. It was a picture of a boy about four years old with his hands and legs tied down to the sides of the chair in which he was sitting. The restraints were needed because the child suffered from Lesch-Nyhan syndrome, a severe X-linked hereditary disorder that leads to a bizarre form of self-mutilation. Because of high acid concentrations in the blood, a boy born with Lesch-Nyhan syndrome will chew compulsively on his fingers and lips until, at a fairly young age, he dies from these and other complications of the disease. Before the child in the picture died, he had bitten off all his fingers and had chewed the tissue from his lower lip all the way down to the tip of his chin. After his death, the family wanted to have another child. Although the mother was Catholic, she had already undergone three abortions of male fetuses in an effort to have a healthy child. Now, following a PGD procedure, she was one month from delivering an unaffected female child. This success was not easily accomplished. No two families with Lesch-Nyhan have exactly the same misspelling among the 57,400 genetic letters that make up the relevant gene. Although it would have been possible to prevent the birth of another child with the disease by selecting only female embryos to transfer, neither the family nor Hughes wanted to discard healthy male embryos. To find embryos free of the mutation, Hughes and his research team had performed a sophisticated genetic analysis. They had only a few hours to do this, between the moment when they took the blastomere for analysis and the time that they had to transfer the healthy embryo back to the womb. PGD, Mark emphasized, is an extremely promising technology with significant moral and psychological advantages over current alternatives. But a great deal of research will have to be done to make it reliable. If such advancements in PGD are made, it may someday be possible not just to discard embryos with genetic defects, but to use gene therapy to alter their genes to correct the genetic errors.

Mark did not emphasize this possibility in his presentation, but we later learned that embryo research is also one of the most promising routes to gene therapy. Many genetic diseases afflict very early fetuses and thus lead to malformed tissues or organs. These developmental problems cannot easily be reversed once the fetus has developed. Because of this, PGD followed by embryonic gene therapy will be a major form of medical intervention in the future. It is somewhat ironic that achieving this goal will require extensive embryo research. Many opponents of embryo research base their views on their opposition to abortion. Yet embryo research is needed if we are to reduce, and perhaps eliminate, the use of abortion for genetic reasons.

Scientific issues continued to dominate the morning's discussion. In light of our goal to articulate a time limit to embryo research, we asked Brigid to give a detailed account of the early stages of embryo development. John Eppig of the Jackson Laboratory in Maine closed the morning with a review of his and others' work. Following Mark Hughes's powerful presentation of clinical research closely linked to the avoidance of serious disease, John's remarks seemed dry and unimportant. His subject was *in vitro* maturation of human oocytes (IVM), a new technology that would permit scientists to gather multiple immature eggs from a woman by a simple in-office procedure and mature them outside her body to the point at which they would be biologically ready for fertilization. If developed, this technology would allow physicians to avoid current regimens that involve injecting women with powerful drugs to make eggs mature within their ovaries. It would also open the door to wholly new sources of donor eggs for reproductive and research purposes. As John methodically clicked through his slides of mouse embryos at different stages of development, it did not really occur to most members of the panel that this technology was the route to major transformations in reproductive medicine. Even less apparent was the fact that John's appeal for increased research in this area would lead to the single most contentious matter before the panel and our most controversial policy recommendation: the issue of "research embryos."

That afternoon's public statements offered a glimpse of the controversies that lay ahead. Several speakers were in favor of embryo research. One woman identified herself as a carrier of fragile X syndrome, a disorder that leads to severe mental retardation. She already had two children who were affected by the disease and had undergone two late-term abortions to prevent the birth of others. Now she urged development of preimplantation genetic diagnosis as an emotionally less traumatic alternative. Several individuals and couples who were struggling with the problem of infertility spoke advocating research in this area. But an increasing number—and soon the majority of speakers at these public presentation sessions—represented an anti-abortion, "pro-life" point of view. Roman Catholic religious publications and those of other anti-abortion organizations had alerted their readers to the panel's existence and had asked them to bring pressure to bear to prevent federal funding of embryo research.

A seemingly innocuous procedural decision by our chairman, Steven Muller, with which we all agreed, did not help matters. It had originally been thought that speakers would be allotted five minutes for their presentation. Then they would be given an additional five minutes to reply to questions from panel members. In response to a request from a speaker, Steven provided the option of using the entire ten minutes for each presentation. The result was a succession of harangues unrelieved by questioning or the opportunity to correct misstatements. Many of these presenters offered a straightforward statement of the "pro-life" position, denouncing all research not of immediate benefit to the embryo. Some were intemperate, invoking images of "bioslavery" and Nazi medical experimentation, or threatening the panel with future Nuremberg-like prosecutions if we helped launch embryo research. At one point during a meeting later in the spring, Steven Muller had enough. A speaker had just finished accusing the panel of unleashing genocide. Growing red in the face, Stephen noted that his own parents had fled Nazi Germany during the 1930s. He was not about to be lectured, he said, by someone who likened him to a Nazi doctor.

One speaker that afternoon, Wendy McGoodwin of the Council for Responsible Genetics, offered objections from a very different point of view. The council was a loose coalition of scientists and others concerned about the possible misuses of genetic research and information. Many of its members, McGoodwin reported, believed that some areas of embryo research were "too ethically and socially problematic to justify federal funding."[159] A major source of concern was preimplantation genetic diagnosis. Council members were worried, she said, that widespread use of this technology "combined with the existing social pressures to create a perfect child, will lead to a kind of commercial eugenics." The council was also concerned about germ-line genetic therapy. She understood that we had been explicitly instructed not to consider this issue in the course of our work. Nevertheless, she reminded us, germ-line therapy will involve the use of embryos because its aim is to alter the targeted gene in every cell of the developing body, which can best be accomplished at the embryonic stage. Unless our panel addressed this issue, she said, it would appear that we had implicitly endorsed what the council regarded as dangerous and unjustified genetic manipulations.

McGoodwin's concerns were arguably removed from the issues facing our panel. To rule out embryo research because in the long run it could lead to genetic abuses seemed neither reasonable nor realistic. PGD was already being developed and applied under private auspices for recognized medical purposes. We could not stop that. A ban on federal involvement might slow research, but it would also guarantee that research (including germ-line research) went on without federal oversight or regulation. Furthermore, it was hard to see how complying with Harold Varmus's request to leave the issue of gene therapy to others amounted to a tacit endorsement of it. McGoodwin's and the council's worries, in other words, were somewhat off the mark insofar as the work of our panel was concerned. But they were significant because they indicated that embryo research faced opposition not from a single camp but from two, diametrically opposed directions. As we had been hearing, embryo research was anathema to large segments of society because it ran counter to their traditional views on prenatal life and abortion. But McGoodwin's presentation indicated that many people on the liberal side of the spectrum of political opinion were also worried about this research. For them it opened the way to the misguided use and commercial exploitation of genetic science. Cultural apprehensions that have existed at least since the publication of *Brave New World* were being stirred. Wendy McGoodwin and the Council for Responsible Genetics did not represent anything like the organized opposition of the "pro-life" presenters. But the fears she expressed were important because they eroded support among informed and socially concerned individuals who normally were a natural constituency in favor of scientific research.

During lunch and the public statements that followed, my mind was on the brief presentation I was to give later that afternoon on the moral status of the human embryo. I had prepared a document in which I tried to translate my basic, choice-based understanding of this issue into a language and set of ideas that would be more appropriate for a public forum and that would also offer a firm basis for the panel's thinking.

When my turn came, I began my remarks with a brief statement about the role of moral theory in helping us think about something as complicated as the status of the human embryo and the protections it might deserve. On the one hand, I noted, there are a series of prevalent beliefs and practices that reflect some of our deepest moral hunches about an issue. These are the "stuff" of moral theorizing, the data we must explain and organize. On the other hand, people put forward a variety of theoretical options as they try to understand the deeper logic of our intuitive moral beliefs and extend them to new and less certain areas of decision. The aim of moral theory, I said, is to arrive at a position in which our most important moral hunches and our formal modes of reasoning fit together. This may require adjusting our theory so that it better explains our most pressing intuitions. Or, we may conclude that some of our intuitively held views are unreasonable and must be rejected. The Harvard philosopher John Rawls, with whom I had studied, used the term "reflective equilibrium" to describe the state in which our theory and most compelling intuitions are in harmony.[160]

This preamble to my remarks was important because I believed the issue of the moral status of the early embryo was badly clouded by too much theorizing. In the course of the debates over abortion, people from all points on the political spectrum had brought their theories to bear on the issue and frequently imposed them on others' moral experience. The impulse was understandable. If any area needed theoretical clarity, it was this one, because, when it comes to the status of nascent life, our intuitions are murky. But too often, theorizing had lost touch with the realities reflected in our most important moral hunches and practices. One very important reality, I knew, was that most people are substantially uninterested in the early embryo, whatever their formal views on abortion. Woman of all religious and moral backgrounds have used the intrauterine device (IUD) for birth control, even though it has long been suspected to work, at least in part, by preventing implantation of fertilized eggs.[161] As I noted earlier, couples involved in IVF procedures routinely consent to making more embryos than can successfully be returned to the womb. No one, in the medical community or elsewhere, expresses concern over the massive loss of life that goes on daily as thousands of embryos, the large majority of all conceptions, fail to implant and are sloughed off. Some may object that people are not concerned about these things because they are unaware of them. But the very lack of awareness suggests disinterest. Can we really believe that once they knew about the massive loss of early embryonic life, citizens would demand a vast, federally funded medical program of embryo rescue? This deep-lying disinterest in the early embryo is telling. Although those who value embryonic life might interpret it as a sign of moral insensitivity or neglect, it suggests to me that much of the concern expressed for the embryo has little intuitive foundation. Instead, it is almost entirely theory-created and theory-driven. It results from poorly developed efforts by ethicists and theologians to undertake the difficult task of conceptualizing life's moral beginning. These efforts lead people to mistakenly mark fertilization as a boundary point in ways that do not harmonize with our most deeply felt intuitions about very early human life and the practices that reflect those intuitions. The challenge now was to indicate, very succinctly, why theorizing about this matter so often goes wrong.

Continuing with my remarks, I noted that in thinking about the status of embryonic human life, we have two broad theoretical approaches available. One may be called the "single criterion" approach. This approach actually comprises many different and sometimes opposing views, but all have one thing in common: proponents "seek out one, or at most a couple, of crucial qualities"[162] that they believe are needed for full moral status. Examples from opposite ends of the spectrum of opinion include those who believe that possession of a new genotype qualifies an entity for full moral protection and those who believe that some sort of developed cognitive status, like self-consciousness or reasoning ability, is needed. Despite the dramatic differences in the moral implications of these views, I said, they share a common theoretical point of departure. Both seek to identify the intrinsic property that makes something a protectable being. Returning to my point about the need for theory to fit our intuitive beliefs, I noted that all of these positions usually end up "being inconsistent with some widespread practices or assumptions that are shared in our society."[163] For example, the view stressing self-awareness or reasoning ability runs directly counter to our very strong commitment to the protection of newborns. The position stressing the genotype runs counter to widespread acceptance of contraceptive methods like the IUD or morning-after pill, which work by preventing implantation.

Against all these "single criterion views," I offered a "pluralistic and pragmatic" approach. What characterizes this approach, I said, is the belief that not one but "a variety of criteria interact and work together to lead to a mounting sense of concern and ultimately to judgments of protectability about entities."[164] I was ready to offer a list of these qualities or criteria. Before doing so, however, I warned that it is a mistake to take any one of them as determinative. A class of beings can lack a quality on the list and still be regarded as deserving protection, or it can possess several qualities and still fail to merit full moral respect. Generally, the greater the number of criteria a class of beings meets, the closer it comes to being fully protectable. In determining the status of a class of beings at a particular stage of development, we have to look at all these qualities and their interrelationships. I could have added that this pluralistic approach is used in other areas of rational choice. We rarely base complex decisions—the choice of a college, a career, a spouse—on a single "necessary and sufficient criterion." Instead, we have a variety of important, intersecting concerns. Our final choice can sometimes involve unexpected emphases—or deletions—from our initial list of desired qualities. The determination of whether a class of beings should be regarded as morally protectable is no different.[165]

I then offered a list of some of the criteria I had in mind. One is developmental potential, a being's likelihood to go on to birth and adulthood. Potential is rarely a complete basis for valuing something, but it does contribute to our judgment when other considerations are present. Another criterion is the semblance of human bodily form. Having a body is important. We respect the body and treat it with reverence even when someone has died. Also important is some degree of developed cognitive ability, although a range exists here, from rudimentary sentience to full self-consciousness and developed rationality. Independent existence is another consideration. The fact that an entity can live on its own and therefore does not physically have to impinge on the life of another person can be an important reason for affording it greater moral weight. Also important are matters that are extrinsic to the class of beings under consideration but that play a role in aiding moral judgment. One example is the fact that a being has passed some critical and easily identified marker event in its development (such as conception, implantation, gastrulation, or birth). The availability of a clear marker might prompt us to regard beings that have passed that point as having reached a stage that warrants more protection.

How did these reflections relate to the panel's task of determining the moral claims of the embryo to research protections? The preimplantation embryo, I observed, possesses at least one of the qualities on this list: a measure of developmental potentiality. This distinguishes it from individual sex cells. But it lacks almost every other quality I indicated. How important is developmental potentiality alone? Probably not important enough, I offered, to justify prohibiting beneficial research. The measure of the early embryo's moral weight, I observed, may be found by looking at other widely accepted practices in society that reflect underlying moral intuitions. I had in mind our general indifference to the early embryo's survival. No practice in our society, I said, suggests that, because of their developmental potential, early embryos have enough claims on us to significantly limit people's ability to pursue important personal or health-related interests. But developmental potential does appear to hold some modest weight. People who work in reproductive medicine laboratories often treat embryos, even those that will not be returned to a womb, differently from other bodily tissues. They may dispose of spare embryos by cremation or other methods used for more developed fetuses. This measure of respect suggests that research should not be left entirely unregulated. I concluded by observing that because some of the qualities on this list, including bodily form and the possibility of sentience, begin to develop with the appearance of the primitive streak at approximately two weeks, good reason exists for selecting this as an important marker event for stricter research limitations.

The "pluralistic and pragmatic" approach I briefly outlined did not emphasize the choice-based nature of these decisions. It bypassed these deeper theoretical matters but tried to concretize their practical import in a series of illustrations of the choice process. Some price was paid for this translation from a rigorous theoretical exposition to a more practically oriented treatment. Months down the line, when the panel's report was finally made public, some writers criticized our handling of the moral status issue. In an article in the *Hastings Center Report,* the center's distinguished bioethicist/director, Daniel Callahan, began on a positive note. "The panel deserves praise," he said, "for the care with which it analyzed the moral status of the preimplantation embryo. No other group has done nearly so well in working its way through that moral thicket." But then he voiced two criticisms. First, he criticized the report for not spelling out the ways in which competing values were to be balanced. Noting that the report accords some moral weight to the preimplantation embryo but does not rule out research, Callahan remarked:

> Though the report sets up a clear moral tension between those two goods, it is utterly silent on how research claims and possibilities should be evaluated for their moral weight and benefit. It is no less silent on how, even with that information in hand, a moral calculus is to be constructed to do the necessary balancing.[166]

In a limited sense, Callahan was right. Neither in my presentation to the panel nor in the section of the report that was eventually based on it did I offer a specific method for making the decision that was thrust on us: to weigh the claims of the preimplantation embryo against the need to conduct potentially important and beneficial research. However, the appropriate method of argumentation was there if one looked carefully. It involved references to other balancing judgments we make concerning the early embryo. This is how I believe we usually proceed in novel deliberative situations. We try to examine related choices we have made in an effort to establish the relative weights of our values. One important area of comparison is with our reproductive behaviors. In the course of infertility procedures, for example, couples of all religious backgrounds routinely create excess embryos that they know will be discarded.[167] These couples apparently believe that the enhanced opportunity of having a child far outweighs the moral worth of individual embryos. This suggested to me that the claims of the embryo were not very great, and probably not great enough to outweigh the value of research aimed at curing or preventing serious diseases.

Callahan's second criticism indicated that he had missed the deeper logic of the pluralistic approach I was offering. I had said, and the final report repeated, that at fourteen days of development, or with the appearance of the primitive streak, the embryo begins to acquire characteristics that make its use in research more questionable. Callahan asked,

> If the emergence of the primitive streak is such a decisive event why then should it not be used to set a limit on abortion as well? Why . . . is it not acceptable to carry out medically enlightening and socially useful research on an embryo after fourteen days, but perfectly acceptable to kill a fetus for any reason a woman privately deems permissible up to twenty-four weeks?[168]

Callahan's question reveals how difficult it is to put to rest the search for the defining characteristic that qualifies an entity for moral protection. I had argued (and the panel later agreed) that what happens at the time of the emergence of the primitive streak is important enough to warrant imposing significantly increased limitations on research. In Callahan's thinking, this translated into acknowledgement of a decisive change in the status of the embryo, the emergence of some new "property" that established its basic protectability. Possession of this "property" also justified prohibiting abortion after this point. "Since the primitive streak is all-important," Callahan seemed to be saying, "how can we permit the destruction for any reason of a later-term fetus that has achieved this stage of development?" What Callahan was missing, however, is the basic insight that these line-drawing efforts are balancing judgments in which we weigh the claims on us of the entity against the impact that protecting it can have on all our liberties. I had argued that the developing qualities in the embryo, when weighed against the likely benefits of research beyond the time of gastrulation, recommended selecting this event as a marker for increased research restrictions. We were balancing the claims of the embryo against our research needs, and the argument was that at this point in the embryo's development, these claims had sufficient weight to recommend restraint. Abortion poses a totally different question. Do the claims of the embryo or fetus at any stage of development take precedence over a woman's freedom to terminate a pregnancy? Freedom to determine what happens to one's body is a liberty interest of undisputed value. Examining this matter in its 1973 *Roe* v. *Wade* decision, the U.S. Supreme Court concluded that a woman's liberty in this area has priority in the first and second trimesters of pregnancy. During the second trimester, a concern for maternal health permits the state to require that abortions be performed in a medical setting. In the third trimester, the developing array of qualities in the fetus creates a substantial state interest in its protection, which may be overridden only to protect a woman's life and health. This sensible, staged, developmental approach is an excellent example of what it means to establish boundary lines and degrees of protection for a class of entities. At each stage, the court weighed the growing magnitude of the fetus's claims on us in relation to the interests of women and society. Our panel was trying to do the same thing with a different set of interests, those related to the early embryo and medical research. We eventually took a fairly cautious position and concluded that after gastrulation the embryo's claims outweighed the benefits of most foreseeable forms of medical research. Callahan interpreted this single complex balancing judgment to represent a change in the embryo itself that was decisive and that applied to all other moral questions that might arise concerning it. His criticism thus embodied what I see as a long history of misapprehending the nature of such boundary determinations. Decisions made for specific types of reasons in specific types of circumstances for an entity with certain characteristics are converted into the belief that any entity with those characteristics merits protection in all circumstances.

Similarly mistaken reasoning has led some people to argue that, because we now make intensive efforts to save the lives of some very premature newborns, the fetus at the same gestational age merits exactly the same degree of protection. Some ask, "Is it not unreasonable to try desperately to save the life of a twenty-four-week gestational age newborn on one floor of the hospital, while permitting the abortion of a same-age fetus on another floor?" This question misses the point that the balancing judgments for prebirth and postbirth infants involve very different considerations. At any fetal age, limiting a woman's right to end a pregnancy imposes serious restraints on her life and liberty. In contrast, sustaining the life of a premature child usually accords with the parents' wishes and the professional commitments of medical caregivers. Refusing to sustain such children when their lives can be saved runs counter to a host of important values. That people miss these distinctions and focus merely on the intrinsic biological similarities between *in utero* fetuses and *ex utero* children at these gestational ages indicates the tenacious hold of the habit of mind that looks only to the entity itself for the defining features of protectability.

Recall that, in my presentation, I had introduced the term *pluralistic* to describe the approach I was advocating. This term has at least several different meanings in this context; my use of it to capture all of them was deliberate. I first meant to suggest that a plurality of considerations is important in determining the status of a class of entities. I was thus renouncing the habit of looking for the single necessary and sufficient condition for the possession of moral status. Second, I was rejecting a definitional route to such conclusions in favor of a choice-based approach that more accurately describes how we think about these matters. Third, I was offering a view on how boundary and status determinations like this should be made in the context of a pluralistic society. The plurality of considerations that indicate when a class of beings should receive moral protection roughly corresponds to the diversity of views on this matter present among members of society. Each quality on this list has its supporters in society's debates over the moral status of prenatal life. Some people emphasize developmental potential alone, believing it sufficient to justify bestowing full protection on the embryo; others hold that sentience is required; and so on. By using the term "pluralistic," I was signaling that no single criterion, no one position, should hold sway in these debates. Each quality has some importance, but only when enough of them are present to compel widespread assent do we approach anything like a reasonable consensus on the embryo's relative value. Only then can we say with confidence that the entity has a strong enough claim on enough of us to merit its being protected at some cost to our liberty. In my remarks to the panel I tried to express this idea by contrasting it with those positions, some of which are influenced by religious beliefs, that take one defining feature of personhood as definitive. "What public policy is about at this point," I said, "is not ultimate metaphysical truths. We are not trying to learn what in God's eyes is personhood. People in our society will differ substantially about their view as to where God believes the unique person commences." In contrast, "we are making an essentially social and public policy decision . . . as to when we're going to intervene and protect." That decision, I concluded, "is made on the basis of this multiplicity of criteria, all of which are reasonable and compelling, and caution restraint when they become significantly present."[169]

I had barely finished speaking when Alta Charo raised her hand to offer an interpretation of my remarks. "If I understand you correctly," she said, the value placed on the embryo "is really determined not by specific criteria that could be applied to determining the inherent value of the embryo, since there's so much disagreement about that, but rather by the value that all of us who have been born and thought about this have placed on the embryo." Understanding her to be trying to express an aspect of my choice-based view, I nodded my head in tentative agreement. Alta continued: "So the concept of respect would be more respect for the moral pain that some people feel at seeing the destruction or frivolous use of embryos; that we shouldn't be talking so much about respect for embryos as much as respect for people who feel strongly about the way embryos are used. . . ." That pain, she added, is real, not symbolic.

"Pain" seemed to me to be too strong a word. "Concern" more accurately describes some people's investment in the embryo, although sometimes people do feel emotional pain when they believe that embryos are being mistreated. But Alta's basic point seemed right. It is not the embryo itself, which is not itself a subject of experiences, that is important here but our various stakes in it. Some of these stakes are direct, such as the emotional attachment some women may feel to a pregnancy beginning within them. Some are conceptual, as when we fear that mistreatment of embryos may lead to other, more serious harms. Some people's stakes are based on imaginative projections but are nonetheless emotionally real for them, as when they regret the loss of a "future life" that might have existed but for a miscarriage or abortion.

Alta concluded by saying "it becomes a question in a pluralistic society of how you balance that kind of moral pain against the specifically articulated guaranteed rights of association, or liberty, or bodily control." I replied by saying that I agreed with this way of putting things. These matters are a social choice. Moved by different concerns, people bring their arguments for protecting a class of beings to all our attention. But every extension of protection must also be measured against its impact on everyone's liberties and welfare.

In the weeks ahead, Alta's voice was one of the strongest raised in defense of attention to women's stakes in our decisions. Alluding at one point to the many thousands of women around the world whose lives and health are jeopardized by unwanted pregnancies, she urged us to adopt the most permissive regulations regarding embryo research in order to promote the development of better contraceptive methods. When the choice was viewed as that between the life and health of adult women and some people's moral concerns for the early embryo, Alta clearly opted for the former. Eventually, the panel probably bowed more to the side of respect for others' moral sensitivities than she would have liked. Our final recommendations placed strict limits on the creation or use of embryos for research purposes. Nevertheless, from this point onward, we consistently adhered to the way of thinking about this issue that I had introduced and that Alta had championed. Respect for the embryo, amounting to respect for qualities it possessed that some people regarded as important, would be weighed against real impacts on people's life and health. In that weighing, people's real and compelling health interests usually took priority.

As clear as this balancing approach seemed to me and, eventually, to other members of the panel, I knew that many people in society would disagree. Some of them arrived at their positions because they adopted a theoretical approach that emphasized one feature of the embryo (genotype or developmental potentiality, for instance) as morally definitive. Others got there because their moral hunches and intuitions led them personally to value early embryos more than the medical benefits of research. How should we respond to those holding these views? Alta had furnished part of the answer. In a pluralistic society, you strive to respect the views of others, including those with whom you disagree. One should try to minimize their moral "pain" as much as possible while not relinquishing vital social objectives. This is particularly true when the use of federal funds is involved, because such funding can (at least financially) involve people against their will in activities with which they morally disagree. Other things being equal, we should avoid governmental support for controversial research and instead seek private funding for it. In my discussion of stem cell research in chapter 7, I will indicate how this reasoning led me to support a position involving federal funding for the use, but not the derivation, of human stem cell lines.

But other things are not always equal. The same balance of considerations led me to a different conclusion regarding the possibility of federally funded embryo research. As an expert panel, the question before us was whether the goals of minimizing the health risks for women and children and fostering beneficial new medical research outweighed the claims of the early embryo. Our answer would be "yes." We also came to believe that federal funding was necessary to stimulate the high-quality research needed to attain these goals. Private clinics financed by revenues lacked the resources for the necessary multicenter studies on the safety and efficacy of new reproductive procedures. They certainly could not fund research on broader issues of embryology and birth defects. We also believed that federal funding would provide more opportunity for ethical oversight of research than would handing it all over to the private sector or overseas researchers. Among other things, it would bring those infertility programs conducting research and utilizing federal funds under the protective umbrella created by existing human subjects regulations.[170] For all of these reasons, we concluded, federal funding was needed. Did it make a difference that millions of Americans disagreed with this conclusion? In political terms it did, because many of these people would certainly try to reverse our judgment through the political process. But the task of a multidisciplinary expert panel like ours was not to count noses. It was to weigh the moral and scientific issues and make recommendations for public policy. Here, respect for the sensitivities of the opponents of embryo research counted less than the people whose lives and health this research could protect.

Most panel members seemed to find my arguments convincing. The approach I offered provided a way to understand why the early embryo has limited claims on us from the perspective of public policy. It also provided some basis for understanding the corresponding increase in concern that accompanies the appearance of the primitive streak. My draft section on this issue eventually went into our final report with few changes. We never again had reason to engage in extended discussion of this issue. With the question of the moral status of the early embryo behind us and the reasoning at hand to justify our position, the panel could turn to more detailed matters.

4

THE ISSUE OF
RESEARCH EMBRYOS

N O question absorbed more of the panel's time or stirred more controversy than whether we would recommend that scientists be allowed to
create embryos solely for research purposes, with no intention of using them
to help establish a pregnancy. Even the choice of language to describe this
possibility was controversial. The word "create" heightened concerns that we
would be seen as allowing scientists to "play God." In the end, we chose the
phrase "fertilization of oocytes expressly for research purposes" and spoke of
"developing research embryos" as distinguished from using "spare embryos"
left over from infertility procedures.

The issue was not new. As early as 1979, the U.S. Ethics Advisory Board
concluded that the creation of research embryos was ethically acceptable in
order to establish the safety of *in vitro* fertilization.[171] Regulations issued by
Britain's Human Fertilisation and Embryology Authority permit the creation
and use of research embryos for a variety of reasons. These include studies
that promote advances in the treatment of infertility, the development of
knowledge of the causes of miscarriages and congenital diseases, contraception research, and research on preimplantation genetic diagnosis (PGD).[172]
The recent Canadian report on new reproductive technologies had recommended that it be legal in Canada.[173] In Europe, the issue was being debated
by the bioethics steering committee of the Council of Europe. Many Euro-

pean bioethics groups opposed the creation of research embryos, and the council's treaty on bioethics eventually banned it.[174] Britain, whose national law preceded the treaty, remains exempt from this provision.

Even though the issue was in the background from the beginning of our work, it grew in importance with each meeting of the panel. A major stimulus to our thinking, although we did not realize it at the time, was John Eppig's presentation at the 4 March meeting. With his overview of research on *in vitro* maturation (IVM) of eggs, John had introduced us to a technology that might transform reproductive medicine. IVM is the key to solving a host of troubling problems in the current practice of assisted reproduction. Two technologies have revolutionized reproductive medicine in recent years. *In vitro* fertilization (IVF) permits clinicians to establish a pregnancy when a woman's fallopian tubes are blocked or missing and also allows women without ovarian function to take advantage of donor eggs. Intracytoplasmic sperm injection (ICSI) helps clinicians overcome many problems of male-factor infertility, from low sperm count to physiological difficulties in sexual functioning. However, both IVF and ICSI require a supply of eggs that are ready for fertilization, and this remains the problem with much reproductive medicine today.

Each month during a woman's fertile years, premature (preantral) ovarian follicles mature under hormonal influence and pass out of her ovaries into her fallopian tubes, where fertilization occurs. Of the estimated supply of one to two million eggs that a baby girl has at birth, only one or two eggs will be ready for fertilization each month when she reaches sexual maturity. In the early years of IVF, dependence on this natural cycle contributed to the low success rate of procedures, since only one or two embryos could be produced for transfer back to the womb. A major breakthrough was the introduction of powerful stimulatory drugs that increased the number of mature (antral) follicles containing ripe eggs. This drug regimen allows clinicians to collect many mature eggs from a woman, fertilize them, and, since there are often more embryos produced than can safely be transferred, freeze the remaining ones for later use. Although drug stimulation adds to the cost of a single IVF cycle, it greatly enhances the overall success of an extended course of treatment.

As any woman who has undergone IVF knows, this regimen is not pleasant. The drugs have powerful physiological and emotional effects, including restlessness, insomnia, nervous tension, depression, and mood swings. These effects sometimes contribute to marital tensions and difficulties that beset couples already struggling with infertility. Because of their effects on the ovaries, women suffering from certain conditions that cause infertility, such as polycystic ovarian disease, cannot use the drugs. As I previously mentioned, they may also have a long-term impact on a woman's health. Published reports to date have offered contradictory evidence as to whether these medications increase the risk of ovarian cancer.[175] The issue will probably not be settled until long-term, multicenter studies are conducted (or, worse, until the current generation of IVF patients begins to experience significant problems). Finally, these drugs may damage the eggs that are produced. This could be a cause of the relatively high rate of implantation failure in IVF, and it may have long-term implications for the health of children produced by assisted reproductive procedures. During the late 1940s and early 1950s many women were prescribed the drug diethylstilbestrol ("DES") to stabilize early pregnancies. It later emerged as a cause of cancer and reproductive system defects in female and, to a lesser extent, male children. Sadly, DES daughters and sons are now disproportionately represented among those using IVF and other assisted reproductive procedures.[176] Although no similar links have been found between the drugs now being used and long-term adverse effects on offspring, history reminds us that the risk exists.

IVM could reduce or eliminate many of these problems. By means of a relatively simple laparoscopic or needle aspiration procedure, it would be possible to remove a large number of immature follicles from a woman's ovaries. Using IVM, these eggs could be matured outside a woman's body, sparing her exposure to stimulatory medications. In time, research might also shed light on the maturation process itself and permit the development and use of improved media for egg maturation, further reducing the risk to any children born. Because many immature eggs can be harvested at once, standard infertility procedures for some women would also make many donor eggs available to women who do not ovulate at all. This might help reduce the controversial practice of paid egg donation that induces many young women donors to subject themselves to high levels of drug stimulation.[177]

IVM is thus a major route to safer and more effective infertility medicine.[178] But its initial development, as John Eppig made clear to us, requires the deliberate fertilization of eggs. To do this work in human beings, one must begin with immature oocytes and bring them up to and through fertilization as a crucial test of their normalcy and developmental competence. By definition, spare embryos, which represent eggs that have already been fertilized, cannot be used for this purpose. Successful procedures must produce eggs that will fertilize and undergo cleavage. Because new, untested procedures and growth media will be involved, it would be irresponsible at the start of this research to return any eggs that have been matured and fertilized in this way to the womb. Doing so would risk the lives and health of any children born and the women who carry them.

This ethical requirement of prior research on embryos not intended for transfer applies to all new assisted reproductive technologies. During the early 1970s, when Robert Steptoe and Patrick Edwards were developing IVF, they initially fertilized a number of human oocytes that were not transferred back to a womb.[179] The conception and birth of Louise Brown in 1978 was thus the end point of their initial research. In chapter 6 I will try to argue that we wrong a future child by carelessness or neglect in our reproductive conduct. For this reason, we have a duty to minimize the health risks to which we expose future children.

The challenge that parents and society face, therefore, is to reduce as much as possible the risks that children are exposed to as a result of the technologies that make their birth possible. In the context of reproductive research, this means first conducting all possible animal research. Where there are limits to this research because animal models either are not available or are inappropriate, it means the creation and use of research embryos before procedures are carried out at the clinical level to establish a pregnancy. Unfortunately, in the last twenty years, this ethical requirement has largely been ignored. Individual practitioners and clinics have introduced novel procedures with little attention to prior testing. Overall, we have been lucky, but there have been some adverse consequences. For example, as I previously indicated,[180] evidence is growing that ICSI increases the chances of birth defects in the resulting children. This risk may be explained by the fact that men who suffer from infertility also have a higher incidence of other chromosomal or genetic problems, or by the possibility that something in the ICSI procedure, especially the direct insertion of major portions of the sperm body into the egg nucleus, has a damaging effect on egg structures. Sustained laboratory research on human embryos before this procedure was clinically implemented could have helped answer these questions.

Any study that begins with gametes or that requires fertilization as an end point necessitates the use of research embryos. A major example is research on contraceptives. The goal is to better understand the complex processes leading to sperm penetration and syngamy and to devise safe and effective ways of interrupting them. Research of this sort cannot possibly involve the use of embryos left over from infertility procedures, because these embryos are already fertilized. It is necessary to start with eggs and sperm. The first test of success or failure is fertilization. The use of novel methods to try to block fertilization also means that it would be unsafe to transfer any embryos that might be created to a womb. Embryos meant for transfer should never be exposed to chemicals aimed at disrupting fertilization. This research must thus begin and end with the intent to discard any resulting embryos.

As Alta Charo repeatedly reminded the panel, the absence of good contraception is a leading health problem all over the world. In poor nations, unwanted pregnancies are a major threat to maternal and child health and often lead to a high rate of illicit abortion, which carries its own serious health effects.[181] In developed countries, the most effective contraceptives, such as the birth control pill and contraceptive implants, are not free of potentially harmful long-term side effects. For decades, Japanese physicians resisted the introduction of the pill into that country partly because of their concerns about its side effects. The result has been one of the highest abortion rates in the world.[182] Research leading to inexpensive contraceptive vaccines or to effective new spermicides that could be used before or after intercourse to block fertilization would be a major step forward in solving these problems. It would also contribute to a reduction in the incidence of abortion, a goal shared by many who otherwise oppose embryo research.

The need to test the agents and growth media used in reproductive procedures is another reason for the need to develop research embryos. Some drugs used in conjunction with reproductive medicine risk not only the women taking them but the eggs and embryos exposed to them. Eggs and embryos are especially sensitive to teratogens, substances that cause stillbirths or birth defects by disrupting genetic or cellular functioning. Even a deficiency of vital nutrients or metabolites can cause severe harm, as the recent discovery of the link between folic acid deficiency and neural tube defects shows. Before significant new agents are introduced for clinical use in reproductive, gynecological, or perinatal medicine, therefore, the responsible thing to do is closely monitor gametes and embryos experimentally exposed to them. The same is true for other drugs that might be used by women who are planning or likely to become pregnant. New anticonvulsive medications intended for use by women suffering from seizure disorders are an example. Currently, many of these women face a terrible choice. They can stop taking their existing medication and risk seizures that can harm them or their fetus, or they can continue to use medications with possible teratogenic effects. More rigorous testing of these drugs with research embryos could expand these women's range of choices.

There is one other major reason why research embryos are needed. Some studies cannot be conducted without a control population of normal, healthy embryos. A high percentage of spare embryos, those remaining from infertility procedures, evidence cytoplasmic, chromosomal, or genetic anomalies. This may be one reason that the couples who donate them experience infertility because, as a rule, damaged embryos are less able to implant. In addition, because these couples are desperately seeking to have a child, they usually donate only the poorest quality embryos, those that their clinicians judge to be unsuitable for transfer. Research based on these embryos can produce seriously misleading conclusions. In studies seeking to understand the role that certain drugs or nutritional deficiencies play in causing birth defects and pediatric cancers, for example, it is difficult to separate the damage inherent in the embryo from that caused by the agents under study. For important basic research on factors affecting embryological development, therefore, a population of normal embryos is sometimes needed.

Besides all these immediate health-related reasons for creating research embryos, one additional research area in which fertilization is the desired outcome came to our attention: the cryopreservation of human oocytes. Like many people, we were surprised to learn that in an era of routine sperm and embryo freezing, human eggs still cannot be frozen. One reason for this is that freezing apparently disturbs the mechanisms that permit sperm penetration of the egg once it is thawed. As the largest cell in the human body, the egg also contains a great deal of water. When it is frozen, crystals tend to form that can damage sensitive cellular structures and DNA. Two other features of the egg cell compound this freezing problem. One is that the zona pellucida resists passage of the cryopreservant agents used to prevent crystallization. The second is that the egg's genetic material is in an unusual state of suspended animation, prophase I of meiosis, that makes it especially vulnerable to damage. In contrast, sperm can be frozen because they are relatively small and pass through meiosis when they are initially formed. The embryo is also relatively resistant to freezing damage because with each cleavage division its cells remain within the fixed perimeter of the zona pellucida and individually reduce in size.

In 1997 a team of researchers at a private Atlanta infertility clinic overcame the first of these problems—the thawed egg's resistance to sperm penetration—by using ICSI to fertilize previously frozen eggs. A twin pregnancy resulted.[183] Despite this accomplishment, the success rates remain very low, and no systematic studies have been done to investigate the safety of this procedure for the resulting children. Once again, assisted reproductive medicine is moving ahead on a clinical basis with little oversight of the long-term safety of its efforts. In Great Britain, where the Human Fertilisation and Embryology Authority (HFEA) provides comprehensive oversight and research support, the freezing of eggs is allowed, but the transfer of frozen eggs to a woman's womb is currently forbidden.[184]

If egg freezing could be routinely accomplished and its safety demonstrated, it would represent a major medical achievement and an important benefit for many women and families. Women undergoing chemotherapy for cancer or similar treatments often experience serious damage to their ovaries and become sterile. Egg freezing would allow those facing this problem who have not yet married or completed their family to store eggs for later use. In the longer term, this technology could help millions of women in modern societies who currently choose to defer childbearing, often to a point at which they experience reproductive difficulties. Because of extended periods of educational preparation and changing cultural norms, many women today do not consider starting a family until well into their thirties. It is unlikely that this career pattern will soon change, but female reproductive physiology was not designed for it. Each passing year of exposure to bodily processes degrades a woman's supply of eggs. This is a major cause of the increased number of birth defects, such as Down syndrome, that occur in children born to older women. It also contributes to the higher rate of infertility in this population. The problem is not primarily the impact of advancing age on the ability of a woman's body to carry a child. Although they require careful monitoring and good obstetrical care, women in their forties can have healthy babies.[185] Rather, the principal problem lies with eggs whose chromosomes degrade with the passage of time. This increases the incidence of both infertility and birth defects.

Egg freezing could change all of this. Once both this technology and IVM are developed, a woman in her teens or twenties could undergo a laparoscopic procedure and put aside a store of immature eggs that could be preserved in a frozen state indefinitely.[186] She might then also have her fallopian tubes tied, providing safe and effective birth control. When she was ready to start a family, some of these eggs could be thawed, brought to maturity by IVM, and fertilized with her partner's sperm. This would require that she undergo an IVF procedure, but since her eggs remain at the chronological age at which they were frozen and since no hormonal stimulation would be needed, this procedure would be far less costly and more reliable than it now is. In this way, women planning to start a family in their mid-thirties or forties could stop "the biological clock." Any children born to them would be as healthy as if they were conceived a decade or two earlier.

For all these reasons, research embryos are the key to a host of important medical and research advances, ranging from those that immediately reduce the dangers of procedures and drugs currently being widely used to those that promise to enhance reproductive options. Several individuals and couples who spoke before our panel said they would be willing to donate gametes for this purpose. The ethical development and use of research embryos requires informed consent by such donors, because no one should be required to participate in any form of embryo research against his or her will or without his or her permission. But assuming that this basic norm is respected, why should we recommend prohibiting couples who are participating in federally funded studies from donating gametes for the creation of research embryos? And why should we prohibit investigators from using federal funds for this purpose?

In the course of dealing with this issue, we soon learned that many people are opposed to the use of research embryos and federal involvement in this area. Most who oppose abortion and view life as beginning at conception vehemently oppose the use of research embryos, though some of these people would permit the use of spare embryos. Less expectedly, many people who place no great moral weight on the early embryo and who readily would permit the use of spare embryos also share the view that the deliberate creation of embryos for research somehow steps over an important moral line. This coincidence of opposition from different points on the moral spectrum makes the issue a daunting one from a public policy perspective. Nevertheless, when we look closely at the arguments of those holding these views, they show themselves to be less than coherent. This prompts the question of whether any position that would distinguish between the use of spare embryos and research embryos is ethically compelling.

Those who hold the view that "life begins at conception" normally oppose all embryo research that does not aim at improving the chances of healthy survival of the embryo under study. For them, research that deliberately harms the embryo or leads to its being discarded amounts to killing a child. This cannot be morally justified even if it yields a great deal of beneficial information. Nevertheless, some that hold this view are drawn to permitting research on embryos that have been created by couples wishing to have a child but that are never used. Perhaps as many as a million of these embryos have been cryopreserved around the world.[187] Common sense suggests that when the donors consent, these embryos should be used for beneficial research rather than simply being thrown away. Someone who holds the view that life begins at conception might try to justify the use of these spare embryos by reasoning in the following way: IVF should never be undertaken unless the physician and couple intend to fertilize only that number of embryos that can safely be returned to a womb. Nevertheless, it is a sad fact of life that this norm is not always respected. As a result, many spare embryos are frozen and, eventually, destroyed. Because these embryos are doomed anyway, it is morally permissible to use them in research that produces significant health benefits. In this way, their existence will not be in vain. It is *always* wrong, however, intentionally to fertilize an egg for research purposes only. This amounts to the deliberate creation and destruction of a human life.

Initially, this position seems plausible. It appears to justify a moral distinction between the use of spare and research embryos, even from an anti-abortion, "pro-life" framework. But, as my panel colleague Carol Tauer has argued, it invites a serious objection.[188] If the early embryo is morally equivalent to any other human being, why should its abandonment and imminent death justify research on it? Vulnerable groups such as condemned prisoners and terminally ill patients are not usually regarded as research subjects. Indeed, they are often accorded special additional research protections.[189] Why should embryos, if they are the moral equals of such persons, be treated differently? As Tauer observes, an appropriate response to an embryo's abandonment would seem to be redoubled efforts to ensure its eventual "adoption" through embryo transfer, not its use in research that will lead to its destruction.

If these criticisms are correct, then it would seem that those who believe that life begins at conception cannot have it both ways. They cannot simultaneously affirm the sanctity of the early embryo while permitting research on spare embryos. They must oppose all research not of benefit to the embryo, whether it is spare or deliberately created. Alternatively, if they continue to believe that spare embryos may be used in research, they may have to reconsider their view of the embryo's moral status. Their intuitive acceptance of the use of spare embryos may reflect the view that embryos are suitable for research while a dying person is not suitable because embryos have a lesser moral status. If this is so, it is reasonable to ask whether the distinction between spare and research embryos is really as important as they believe. If the moral claims of embryos have less weight than do those of children or adults, why is it wrong to create embryos for research purposes when, by doing so, we can significantly benefit living people?

Some who do not believe that life (morally) begins at conception and accord much less moral weight to the early embryo have also defended a distinction between spare and research embryos. Those holding this view usually think that clinicians are justified in producing many more embryos than are needed for transfer in order to help a couple start a pregnancy. They have no moral qualms about not transferring embryos that show any sign of abnormality. In view of this willingness to subordinate the embryo to considerations of people's reproductive needs, why do they then oppose the creation and use of research embryos when significant medical benefits to living people might result?

The principal argument here is a symbolic one. Although these people do not regard the embryo itself as a research subject that can be injured, they nevertheless believe that its mistreatment can have a serious impact on our respect for the sanctity of life. Research with spare embryos under stringently controlled conditions does not jeopardize this respect, they contend. By enhancing human health and welfare, this research may even reinforce humanist values. But deliberately creating embryos for research purposes goes too far. The philosopher Kant offered a key principle of ethics that states that every human being must be treated not merely as a means but as an end in itself.[190] Even though the early embryo may not be a human being in a strict moral sense, creating and destroying it in research contexts *appears* to constitute using it merely as a means and seems to violate Kant's principle.

In May 1996, in a *New England Journal of Medicine* "Sounding Board" opinion column critical of the panel's report, George Annas, Arthur Caplan, and Sherman Elias offered an additional argument against the creation of research embryos.[191] They maintained that it is the parents' procreative intent that justifies creation of embryos in assisted reproduction procedures. Sundered from that intent, however, the creation of embryos is morally repugnant:

If two people seek to have a child and create a number of embryos to help them do so, there can be no doubt that they hope that at least one of those embryos will become a child. For most people it is the intention to create a child that makes the creation of an embryo a moral act. To create embryos solely for research—or to sell them, or to use them in toxicity testing—seems morally wrong because it seems to cheapen the act of procreation and turn embryos into commodities.[192]

In 1999, the National Bioethics Advisory Commission (NBAC) returned to Annas, Caplan, and Elias's argument in the context of a draft of its report on stem cell research. As we will see in chapter 7, the matter of research embryos has once again become critical, since the possibility of creating autologous (immune system compatible) stem cell lines for tissue repair may require the deliberate creation of embryos for this nonreproductive purpose. Although the NBAC did not ultimately recommend the use of research embryos for this purpose, the draft report found the three authors' argument unconvincing. "The problem with this intuition," the draft observed, "is that it is difficult to see what the intention of the maker of something has to do with the moral status of that thing once it has come into being. We do not think, for example, that the moral status of children is a function of their parents' intention at the time of conception."[193]

This discussion was eventually dropped from the final NBAC stem cell report.[194] The NBAC commissioners ultimately based their opposition to the creation of research embryos largely on symbolic grounds, especially on concerns over the instrumentalization and commodification of human life. In my view, these concerns also explain the force of Annas, Caplan, and Elias's misleading argument. It is not really the embryo that is at issue. What worries us is the impact of these practices on our respect for human life. Where a "good" (procreative) intent is present, we permit a variety of practices, including the creation of excess embryos and their eventual discard or use in research. Where a less good or bad ("mere research") intent is present, we hesitate, fearing the message sent about human life and the moral callousing we might foster.

During and after the panel's deliberations, this essentially symbolic argument was repeated in many forms in scholarly journals and the press. Like all symbolic arguments used in moral contexts, however, it rests on a series of either debatable or speculative assumptions. One is that research is somehow a less worthy purpose than human procreation and thus requires much more justification than does helping couples have children. This view may be shaped by the history of past research abuses or by the belief that research serves only commercial purposes. However, it ignores the value of research in contributing even to the acknowledged aim of assisting families in their reproductive efforts. Good reproductive research using research embryos can make it possible for couples to have children. It can also contribute to the cure of many life-threatening diseases. Why should the pursuit of these goals be thought to cheapen human life? In chapter 7 I will suggest that when stem cell research requiring the use of research embryos reaches the point of promising real cures, the hesitancy about research embryos will subside. Unfortunately, it may be that sustained attention to all the issues surrounding research embryos will have to be postponed until that time.

Those who employ these symbolic arguments also believe there is a real connection between the instrumentalization they perceive in the use of research embryos and a diminished respect for human life. But there is no evidence for this connection. British law has formally permitted the creation of research embryos in governmentally supported programs since the early 1990s. Nothing suggests that British attitudes or conduct have been affected. Symbolic arguments like this have emotional force but are typically hard to substantiate.

Given the stakes, some that find this symbolic argument persuasive urge caution. Where something as important as our respect for the sanctity of human life is concerned, they say, we should move slowly and permit research innovations only when we are confident they will not lead to dehumanization. But how do we balance this caution against the immediate needs of people whose health is jeopardized by poorly researched medical procedures? As a panel charged with shaping the course of research in reproductive medicine, the interests of identifiable constituencies were also on our minds. How do we evaluate the health of women currently being exposed to the risk of cancer because a research ban has slowed development of safer alternatives to stimulatory drugs? How do we balance symbolic concerns against the harms done to a generation of babies born as a result of poorly researched and risky reproductive procedures? How do we weigh the ongoing burden for the millions of women who are deprived of adequate contraception against symbolic worries about the implications of research embryos?

A sign of how difficult we found this issue is that debate about it occupied a major portion of our meetings in April, May, and June. Among the panelists, policy co-chair Pat King took the lead in raising questions about the wisdom of permitting the creation of research embryos. Pat was a veteran of federal bioethics panels, having served during the 1980s as a member of the President's Commission for the Study of Ethical Problems in Medicine and Biomedical and Behavioral Research. A lawyer and professor at Georgetown University Law Center, Pat was more sensitive to the public's response to an expert commission's work than were others on the panel, although Ken Ryan, who chaired the earlier National Commission for the Protection of Human Subjects of Biomedical and Behavioral Research, evidenced his commitment to reproductive medicine by strongly opposing Pat on this matter. Pat articulated several worries. On a personal and ethical basis, she was disturbed by the means-ends reasoning that underlay any proposal for the creation of research embryos. Such reasoning, she pointed out, could also be used to justify beneficial research on the mentally disabled or otherwise vulnerable groups of subjects.[195] From a public policy perspective, she was worried about undermining the credibility of the panel's other, more conservative recommendations. During our 11 April meeting, Pat voiced this concern: "One of the things I'm finding very troublesome in this discussion . . . as somebody that's laboring in the vineyards and has watched all this stuff, fetal research, go on for the last twenty years, is that we want to accomplish it all in one fell swoop."[196] Pat's concern was shared by Bernie Lo, who urged putting the research embryo issue aside for the time being until the public became comfortable with more limited research using spare embryos.[197]

As an African American woman, Pat also worried about the special impact on poor minority women if federal funds were used to pay for eggs donated for research purposes only. Currently, most paid egg donation involves young, college-educated women who are regarded as attractive donors from the point of view of affluent couples who wish to have babies like themselves. Many sensationalist and some spurious press reports have appeared of couples paying outlandish sums to college students or models for egg donation.[198] But if the federal government were allowed to fund the creation of research embryos, poor African American women, who would not ordinarily be approached as donors, would become a natural population on which to draw. They might be attracted even by modest payments, and, provided that they did not suffer from a genetic disorder, their eggs would be suitable for research. Not only would this pattern of donation have an unsavory appearance in terms of the commodification of poor people's reproductive capacity, it would expose these women to stimulatory regimens with unknown long-term risks. In Pat's eyes, federal support for the creation of research embryos, coupled with payments to women providing eggs, would further exploit a population whose reproductive potential, from slavery onward, had already been much abused.

This last concern of Pat's was widely shared by most other panel members. In order to avoid the creation of a federally supported market in this area, we eventually recommended prohibiting payment for eggs, sperm, or embryos used in federal research. In some ways, this was a more stringent ban than obtained in much other federally sponsored research, where subject-volunteers may receive payment for undergoing a variety of risky procedures, ranging from Phase I safety trials of new drugs to cardiac catheterization. Nevertheless, we were disturbed by the thought that federal funding could stimulate a large market in gametes or embryos as well as the fact that this could disproportionately involve poor people or minorities. Testimony by infertile couples reinforced our confidence that enough genuine volunteer donors could be found. Once IVM was developed and ovarian tissues remaining from surgical procedures could be used as a source of immature eggs, a large supply of donated oocytes would exist for research purposes. Together, these considerations supported our recommendation for a ban on payment.

Pat's other worries were less easily addressed. Although her ethical and political concerns were substantial, she recognized the importance of some research requiring the deliberate fertilization of oocytes. This led her to support permission to create embryos when the research could not otherwise be conducted on spare embryos. This included research on IVM, cryopreservation, and contraception, all of which required fertilization and the monitoring of early development with no intent to transfer. But Pat dug in her heels when any wider use was proposed. She was especially unhappy with any permission based merely on an inadequate supply of embryos for research. In Pat's words, permitting the creation of research embryos just because an insufficient number of spare embryos were available would open the door "willy-nilly" to the uncontrolled generation of life in the laboratory, something she opposed both ethically and politically.

No one on the panel championed the uncontrolled creation of research embryos. If this were allowed, and if an adequate supply of maturable eggs could be secured, human embryos would become a research model of choice. They might then be used in all sorts of less important biomedical contexts, ranging from routine drug toxicology studies to safety tests of cosmetics. Taking into account merely the fact that many citizens would be deeply offended by the use of federal funds for these purposes, no one on the panel wanted to open the doors this wide. Nevertheless, there were compelling reasons for permitting the creation of research embryos, even when the research (as in the case of IVM, cryopreservation, or contraception) did not require fertilization as its end point. Since many spare embryos are of uncertain quality, research based on them would often be of questionable value. Here, the debate became a face-off between Pat King and Brigid Hogan. Brigid, true to her scientific vocation, insisted that the greatest respect that could be shown the embryo was to conduct research on it that is important and valid. Research validity, she insisted, required adequate controls.[199] In studies of sufficient importance, such as efforts to understand the causes of birth defects or pediatric cancers, this meant having available a population of normal embryos, and this meant research embryos.

In the course of these discussions, Brigid pointed out one pragmatic reason for not barring scientists from creating research embryos for important studies such as these. If we insist that only spare embryos be used, she noted, we create an inducement for researchers to exploit some women participating in infertility programs by surreptitiously administering additional hormone stimulation to them. Extra "spare" embryos produced in this way might then be diverted to research.[200] Nan Keohane worried that, at least in the near future, the supply of good quality spare embryos might be reduced as research enhances the ability to pinpoint viable eggs or embryos and reduces the need to stimulate women to produce many surplus eggs.[201] Alta Charo added the observation that a couple's open and informed consent to offer gametes expressly for research purposes might be preferable to after-the-fact consent by couples donating embryos remaining from their efforts to start a pregnancy. These couples, she observed, are struggling with infertility and are often psychologically more vulnerable and distressed than gamete donors who knowingly choose to assist researchers.[202] Alta worried that infertile couples who donated leftover embryos might later come to regret their decision.

These debates dominated our April and May meetings. A straw poll at the end of the 3 May meeting indicated overwhelming support among the panelists for a recommendation that the NIH be permitted to fund research involving the deliberate fertilization of oocytes. Pat King supported this recommendation under only one condition: that funding be limited to research that required fertilization as a necessary end point. The phrasing eventually used was that the research "could not otherwise be validly accomplished." Pat would go no further. Brigid and others continued to press for a slightly broader permission that would permit the deliberate creation of embryos for research of great value requiring the use of control populations. In our report, this eventually took the form of a second condition permitting the creation of research embryos "when a compelling case can be made that this is necessary for the validity of a study that is potentially of outstanding scientific and therapeutic value." In the end, those of us who favored inclusion of this additional condition prevailed. We would permit development of research embryos under these two conditions. In a brief appendix to the final report, Pat articulated her disagreement. The goal of establishing scientific validity by using gametes from "normal" controls, she said, does not provide "a compelling reason to permit the fertilization of oocytes expressly for research." The public, she believed, would not understand this rationale. She also expressed doubt about the argument that spare embryos generated by couples undergoing infertility treatments cannot be used for validation purposes. In any case, she added, this reasoning "carries us perilously close to fertilizing oocytes for no other reason than a scarcity of spare embryos."[203]

Pat's dissent reflected a reasonable disagreement with Brigid's (and the panel majority's) position. The development and use of research embryos was warranted, but lines had to be drawn. Why not draw one at the point where a solid public case could be made that a whole class of research could not otherwise be conducted? Although Brigid wanted to extend this permission to instances in which a compelling case could be made for a control population of embryos, how would this line be sustained by institutional review boards (IRBs) and others faced with inevitable pressure from researchers eager to pursue their work? Throughout these discussions, I found myself listening closely to Pat's remarks and sometimes sharing her concerns. In the end, like most of the others on the panel, I concluded that the health of women and children took precedence. I also felt that the NIH grant review process could support the judgments of research importance that our second condition required. IRBs already made such judgments when they applied federal regulations governing research on children. In cases in which there is no direct benefit to a child and that involve a minor increase over minimal risk, IRBs are asked to determine whether the research is likely to yield "generalizable knowledge . . . of vital importance for the understanding or amelioration of the subjects' disorder or condition."[204] Since IRBs are now making these kinds of decisions, it seemed fair to believe that they could make similar judgments on embryo research.

As I look back now on these debates, I am struck by their multiple ironies. In one respect, Pat, Bernie, and other members of the panel who opposed our moving in this direction were right. The issue did galvanize opposition to our work. Most public reaction in the weeks and months after the publication of our report in late September of 1994 focused on this issue. Nevertheless, it is by no means clear that the fine distinctions Pat urged would have alleviated the problem. Those who opposed the creation of research embryos would not permit *any* creation of embryos for research purposes. There is no reason to believe that Pat's careful distinctions would have impressed them.

A further irony is that, despite the panel's focus on this issue, we missed some interesting ways of approaching it that might have enhanced support for our position. During the 3 May meeting John Eppig introduced an idea in a casual remark that went over all our heads. Although John's descriptions of the importance of IVM research had given impetus to our involvement with this issue, he became increasingly wary as the debate proceeded. Like Pat and Bernie, he worried about the public response to our proposals. At one point, after suggesting that we limit the use of research embryos to the kinds of research requiring fertilization, he added, half jokingly, that maybe we should call such research "syngamy interruptus." No one picked up on it, but the suggestion implicit in this jest contained a good deal of insight. At least some of the research that we felt should be pursued in the near future was aimed at understanding fertilization. We could describe the practice geared toward this aim in several ways. We could call it, as we did, the "development of embryos expressly for research." Or we could describe it as "research on gametes having fertilization as its end point." Both were accurate descriptions, but the latter took the focus off the embryo and its fate and concentrated it on the fact that the research at issue was largely sex cell research.

Alternatively, we could have followed the path of legislators in Victoria, Australia, who, despite their ban on embryo research, maintained the limited possibility of some contraceptive research by defining syngamy as the event bringing the embryo into existence. Within this paradigm, research aimed at preventing sperm penetration of the egg was not "embryo research."

In ethical and policy discussions, the way things are described can be important. I am reminded of a comment by Howard Jones during a lecture he delivered at Dartmouth in our course on assisted reproduction. Jones is the pioneer physician and researcher in reproductive medicine whose Norfolk, Virginia, clinic first introduced many of the new assisted reproductive technologies to the United States. Noting that IVF has never been a popular therapy with state legislators or insurers, Jones asked whether things would have been different if it had initially been called "tubal bypass." This at least would have had the merit of highlighting the possible discrimination in our high social investment in cardiac surgery and near neglect of reproductive medicine. Would a similar approach have expedited acceptance of our recommendation regarding research embryos? Possibly, but the problems were obvious. To follow the path set by the Australians would have been easy, but it would also have ruled out most of the research we had considered, because this required following the egg up to and through syngamy into its earliest cleavage stages. To alter terminology so as to focus on sex cells might have helped, but I doubt that the harshest opponents of our recommendation would have been appeased. They would still have drawn the conclusion that we were permitting the deliberate creation of human embryos and would have marshaled opposition accordingly.

Nevertheless, with the benefit of hindsight, I think we should have followed Pat and Bernie's counsel, modified by John Eppig's terminological recommendation. For the immediate future, we should have recommended permitting research using spare embryos, but also research on gametes "when the necessary end point is fertilization and initial development." This language had the advantage of making very clear why we were permitting research of this sort and would have directly served the purpose of educating the public. We should then perhaps have placed the slightly broader research requiring normal controls in our intermediate category of "warranting further review." This would have afforded the NIH several years of experience in supporting research of this sort. As the benefits of the research materialized, it might also have made possible a broadening of the permission to encompass the use of research embryos as controls. In chapter 7 I will describe my efforts to defend a similarly "incremental" approach to stem cell research when I recount my experiences as a member of an American Academy for the Advancement of Science working group. Once burned, twice shy.

Hindsight is always 20/20. As we will see, after November of 1994, nothing we could have done would have altered the fate of our recommendations. A further irony illustrates this fact. One of the reasons John Eppig moved somewhat to the conservative side in the course of our discussions was his belief that at least some of the research on IVM that he advocated could be conducted on parthenotes. These are mature eggs artificially stimulated to start dividing by an electric shock or by exposure to a solution containing salt or alcohol. Because, as noted, the first several cleavage stages in an embryo are entirely controlled by maternal genes and egg cytoplasm, parthenotes are good models for some studies of early development. In some lower species, like frogs, parthenotes can be brought to advanced stages of fetal development. In mammals, in whom the paternally imprinted genes provided by the sperm are crucial for the development of the placenta, development always stops. No scientific basis exists for thinking that human parthenotes would ever develop beyond the earliest cleavage stages.

Whether we would recommend federal funding for research on parthenogenesis was one of the questions before us. We learned that some proposals of this sort were already in the NIH grant review pipeline. It soon became clear to all of us that such research should be allowed. Not only are parthenotes excellent research models for early development, but parthenogenesis also sometimes occurs spontaneously in women's ovaries, leading to the development of what are called "dermoid cysts." In older women these cysts are not usually life threatening, but in younger women they can develop into malignant tumors. Understanding why parthenogenesis occurs is thus of immediate medical importance. We were aware of popular fears that, once developed, parthenogenesis might produce a race of Amazons able to reproduce without the benefit of men. Substantial religious sensitivity also exists about the concept of virgin birth. But no such things are possible from a scientific point of view, and because the egg at any stage is merely a sex cell on which federally sponsored research has long been performed, we could see no reason to oppose funding for research in this area. The very purpose of an expert panel, we believed, was to sift fact from fiction and to represent the real interests of people in medical research. To oppose parthenogenesis research on the grounds of some expected popular opposition would be to abandon our responsibility.

Expecting that this recommendation would not prove controversial and would eventually take effect, John recommended forgoing some types of embryo research that could be done on parthenotes instead. In the end, even this expectation was disappointed. Parthenogenesis was one of the categories of research for which the new conservative Congress eventually decided to deny funding. This result highlights the difficulty that arises when members of an expert panel try to reason with an eye to the political process. Had we let political considerations guide us, we might have moderated our support of research embryos and emphasized parthenote research. Or we might have pressed our commitment to research embryo funding and backed away from parthenogenesis research. Either move would have distorted our contribution to the public understanding of these issues. Yet, in the end, both areas suffered political failure. This suggests to me that an expert panel works best when it resists the siren call of political efficacy and strives merely to achieve clarity in its scientific, ethical, and policy recommendations. I will return to this theme in Chapter 6 when I compare the work of our panel with the National Bioethics Advisory Commission's report on cloning.

5

POLITICS INTRUDES

═══════════════════════════

T HE final working sessions of the Human Embryo Research Panel took
place on 21 and 22 June 1994. Bethesda had grown hot and humid, and
I welcomed the cool air of the hotel function room. As I negotiated my way
past the usual swarm of spectators and press and took my seat at the center
table, I found a small stack of papers. The top page read, *"The Michael Fund
et al.* v. *Ronald M. Green."* With a start, I realized I was being sued.

Other panel members had similarly personalized copies of the lawsuit at
their places. Donna Shalala, secretary of health and human services, and
Harold Varmus were also named as defendants. Skimming the pages quickly,
I learned that the Michael Fund was named after Michael Policastro, a
twenty-four-year-old Pennsylvania man with Down syndrome. The fund described itself as dedicated to sponsoring research on the causes, diagnosis,
and treatment of Down syndrome. The lawsuit called for an injunction to halt
the panel's work. It alleged, among other things, that the appointment process
for the panel violated federal conflict of interest rules because ten members
of the panel (mostly the scientists) were recipients of NIH grants. It also
argued that federal funding for embryo research would injure Michael Policastro and others with Down syndrome by diverting resources away from
research on their condition. Later, perhaps recognizing that these were tenuous grounds for mounting a lawsuit, the fund added as a plaintiff "Mary

Doe," described as one of the approximately "20,000 human embryos in be-ing, stored in a state of cryopreservation in the *in vitro* labs of this nation." The panel's deliberations threatened Mary's "very life and right to privacy and bodily integrity," the amended lawsuit alleged.

If it had not represented a personal threat, I would have found this suit amusing. The idea that any group of citizens could halt government research because they believed it did not directly benefit them could have the effect of bringing most research to a halt. The suit also evidenced a profound misun-derstanding of the ways in which basic scientific knowledge about human embryology might eventually benefit those with chromosomal abnormalities. Most preposterous was the construal of cryopreserved embryos as litigants and the Michael Fund as their protector. Where were the parents of these alleged "victims" of NIH abuse? How could NIH-funded research be seen as threatening to them when most were destined to be thawed and discarded? If the representatives of the Michael Fund ever considered these questions, that did not seem to give them pause. These people lived in a moral universe where frozen four or eight cell embryos were "preborn children." Their champion was the French geneticist Jerome LeJeune, whose testimony in the Tennessee case of *Davis* v. *Davis* was appended to the lawsuit.[205] He believed that cryopreservation of embryos amounts to genocide. Placed in canisters of liquid nitrogen, deprived of the "warmth" of their mother's womb, these tiny beings, said LeJeune, are consigned to "the concentration can."[206]

Someday, cultural historians will look back and wonder how forces in American society led to such flights of moral fancy. The treatment of prenatal life is an important moral issue, but to liken cryopreserved embryos to small Jewish children behind barbed wire in Nazi concentration camps is not just silly, it is an insult to the memory of the real children who suffered those horrors. In the future, we will have to look back and try to understand how careless thinking, misguided sentimentality, and complex social agendas led people into such moral excesses.

By mid-September, a federal district court judge dismissed the suit, primar-ily on the grounds that embryos are not persons capable of being litigants in U.S. law. On that June morning, however, even this frivolous threat stirred concern among panel members. It was not immediately clear whether the NIH would—or could—defend us. Over lunch we wondered whether we should each seek private counsel. The lawsuit was also part of an increasingly strident series of attacks on the panel and its individual members. A few weeks earlier, each of us had begun receiving gruesome color postcards de-picting a mutilated fetus. The American Life League, an anti-abortion group, sponsored this campaign, which confused fetal tissue and embryo research. Many of the messages written on the postcards offered prayers for our souls and implored us to halt our "research activities." Some of the messages could be interpreted as threats. "We know who you are," read one. These threats were only the beginning. Several years after my service on the panel, I would still receive mail quoting things I said while serving on the panel and listing my name among a group of "assassination targets." In an atmosphere of abortion clinic bombings, the panel seemed an obvious target for disruption or violence. Two security guards were now routinely posted at the entrance of the meeting room.

Focusing on these immediate threats, most of us paid little attention to another document that was included in the materials for the June meeting: a copy of a letter to Harold Varmus signed by thirty-five members of the House of Representatives. The letter expressed concern that the 1993 NIH Revitalization Act, which had eliminated the requirement for ethical advisory board review of human embryo research, was being interpreted by the NIH, among other things, as permitting research on the use of aborted fetuses as egg donors, parthenogenesis, and cloning. It went on to pose other research-related questions as well as questions about how panel members were appointed and what kinds of conflicts of interest might be skewing our work. None of these questions was new. Some of the text in the letter appeared to be borrowed from published articles by Richard Doerflinger of the Catholic Secretariat for Pro-Life Activities, a sign that opponents of our work had friends in Congress. That morning, the letter seemed the least of our worries. We knew it represented a minority perspective and assumed that Congress was unlikely to retreat from the commitment to enhanced reproductive research and freedom that the Clinton administration had ushered in the year before. This was an error. In terms of overall impact on our effort, this letter dwarfed in importance any of the lawsuits or threats we received. Among the signatories was the usual roster of anti-abortion congressmen: Robert K. Dornan, Henry Hyde, Charles Canady, and Rick Santorum. One signatory, however, was Newt Gingrich. In November he would become the leader of the new Republican majority in the House of Representatives.

Drafts of most chapters of our report had been completed by then. When we began our work in January, we had hoped to have a completed report ready in time for the June meeting of the Advisory Committee to the Director of the NIH, but the sheer complexity of our task made that impossible. Now we were aiming for the Committee's December meeting. This meant that a published report needed to be available by September in order to allow members of the Committee and others time to respond. At the outset of our work, Harold Varmus had asked us to place types of embryo research into three categories: acceptable for NIH funding, unacceptable, and warranting additional review. We spent the June meeting debating the meaning of these categories and assigning types of research to one category or another. Although later discussions and votes by fax and e-mail would lead to some minor changes, we were now nearing an agreement on our recommendations. Science writer Kathi Hanna would use the summer to prepare the final report.

As important as our recommendations themselves was the reasoning behind them. We had arrived at three considerations that we believed justified some uses of the *ex utero* human embryo in research. First was the promise of significant human benefit. As stated in the final report, research on the human embryo carries "great potential benefit to infertile couples, families with genetic conditions, and individuals and families in need of effective therapies for a variety of diseases."[207] A second consideration was our assessment of the moral status of the early *ex utero* embryo itself. In the words of the report, "Although the preimplantation human embryo warrants serious moral consideration as a developing form of human life it does not have the same moral status as infants and children." We supported this conclusion by pointing to "the absence of developmental individuation in the preimplantation embryo," its "lack of even the possibility of sentience and most other qualities considered relevant to the moral status of persons," and its "very high rate of natural mortality."[208] This wording reflects the pluralistic approach that I had offered to the panel and that would be developed in chapter 3 of our report.

Finally, we argued, it is better to accomplish federal regulation of embryo research through the NIH funding process than to leave this whole area in the hands of privately funded investigators or clinics. "In the continued absence of federal funding and regulation in this area," we noted, "human embryo research which has been and is being conducted without federal funding and regulation would continue, without consistent ethical and scientific review."

This was one of our most important points. Many people believe that withholding federal funding from an ethically troubling research area brings work in that area to a halt. But the opposite is often true. The fifteen-year-long de facto moratorium had not stopped infertility medicine or embryo research. These continued in private clinics and laboratories around the country. Rather, it had ensured that what research did take place proceeded without the ethical and legal protections afforded by the federal funding process. These include strenuous peer review of the science of each proposal. Lack of peer review is one reason why much of the science in reproductive medicine, as Jonathan Van Blerkom noted, is of questionable quality. Furthermore, federally funded researchers must adhere to strict federal regulations that protect human subjects. This requirement entails detailed review of proposals by local institutional review boards, the membership of which includes scientific professionals, ethicists, and community representatives. Far from facilitating irresponsible research, federal funding intensifies oversight and control.

There is a larger lesson here. One of the distinctive features of the U.S., as compared to the European, approach to regulating biomedical research is the relatively decentralized nature of the system. European countries tend to respond to new and troubling issues in biomedicine by passing legislation that prohibits or strictly regulates forms of research or clinical activities. Britain's Human Fertilisation and Embryology Act, with its detailed provisions governing infertility clinics, embryo research, and human cloning, is an example. The bioethics regulations that came out of the European Parliament's Convention on Bioethics is another. Even though Britain's legislation is considerably more permissive of embryo research than the European Parliament's, both represent "top-down" legislative approaches that formally prohibit researchers or clinicians from conducting specific activities.

The United States, in contrast, relies less on the stick than the carrot, and its system of regulation is highly decentralized and multifaceted. Instead of passing national laws prohibiting activities, the federal government holds out the *conditional* offer of financial support. One condition that must be met is adherence to the federal regulatory process, including its ethical requirements. This approach has several advantages. It never entirely forecloses a line of research that attracts the interests of researchers, clinicians, or patients. Research that intrigues some investigators or that has underlying social support can proceed without federal funding. If it proves to be valuable over time, it can reinsert itself into the federal funding system. This is exactly what is happening now with infertility medicine. The same thing would eventually occur in the area of stem cell research, as privately funded researchers made gains that drew national attention. In this respect, the U.S. approach is more supportive of academic freedom in that it rarely intrudes on scientists' choices of research directions. It is also less obstructive to biomedical innovation, because no one can confidently predict in advance which lines of inquiry will prove most fruitful. Speaking in another context, Alta Charo articulated the difference between Europe and the United States: "The European system tries to design the dog and let it wag its tail. We have 50 or 100 or 150 wagging tails from which we then try to reconstruct our dog."[209]

A second advantage of this approach is that it invites the cooperation of the best scientists and insures that the most advanced, cutting-edge work is under ethical review. A more prohibitory stance can drive research or clinical activities "underground," "offshore," or into the hands of less scrupulous or competent practitioners. The announcement by Richard Seed that he would undertake human cloning experiments no matter what legislative attempts were made to ban them is an example. A physicist with no experience in reproductive medicine, Seed is one of the people least qualified to pursue this line of research.

Finally, the U.S. approach has the advantage of being well suited to a culture like ours that is torn between conflicting philosophical and religious visions about biomedical issues. Given our extreme differences of opinion on matters relating to the beginning and end of life and genetic interventions, a centralized, law-based system of research regulation would inevitably become hostage to our political differences. Power would fall disproportionately into the hands of dedicated minority groups with a strong, single-minded point of view on any issue. The history of fetal tissue and embryo research had shown that even a centralized funding system is not immune to these forces. How much worse would matters be if opponents could totally ban reproductive research?

Against this background, we were ready to vote areas of research into our three categories. (See Appendix B for a listing.) The first category, "acceptable for NIH funding," was essentially open-ended. It included all research on the human embryo not explicitly identified in the report as prohibited or warranting additional review. The final report offered examples of the kinds of research that fit this category. They included studies aimed at improving the likelihood of a successful outcome for a pregnancy; research on the process of fertilization; studies of egg activation and the relative role of paternally derived and maternally derived genetic material in embryo development (which might include parthenogenesis without transfer); and studies of oocyte maturation or freezing followed by fertilization (without transfer) to determine developmental and chromosomal normality. As this last example makes clear, we were prepared to place the creation of research embryos in the permissible category when two conditions were met: (1) "when the research by its very nature cannot otherwise be validly conducted" and (2) "where this is necessary for the validity of a study that is potentially of outstanding scientific and therapeutic value."

The final report also offered a set of basic principles to govern all permissible research. Some of these principles reflected the balance we were trying to achieve between permitting research and respecting the moral significance of the embryo as a developing form of human life. They included the requirement that the research be scientifically valid and likely to produce scientific or clinical benefit; that it be conducted, after passing IRB review, by scientifically qualified individuals in an appropriate research setting; that appropriate prior studies using animals or unfertilized human gametes had been done; that the number of embryos used be kept to the minimum needed for the scientific validity of the study; and that the duration of studies be kept as short as possible. We also insisted on a fourteen-day limit for all research, but permitted an exception just beyond that for research that aimed at reliably identifying in the laboratory the appearance of the primitive streak.

Additional principles reflected our concern for the adult human subjects most immediately affected by research: the donors of gametes or embryos used in research protocols. These principles sought to protect them by a requirement of full disclosure of what would be done with their sex cells or embryos and by the requirement of consent, not just to embryo research in general, but to the specific study in which they were being asked to participate. To prevent donors from being exposed to undue pressure, we prohibited payment for gametes or embryos in federally funded studies or the promise of discounted rates in clinical infertility procedures.[210] Consistent with general NIH principles, we also insisted on the equitable selection of donors and efforts to ensure that benefits and risks were fairly distributed among subgroups of the population. It would be unacceptable, for example, if poor individuals who were least likely to use infertility procedures became the major population of research participants.

Eventually, an entire chapter of the final report (chapter 4) would be devoted to a discussion of donor issues and sources of gametes and embryos for donation. Recognizing that egg retrieval procedures required the administration of high doses of stimulatory medications, we asked that women not already involved in a fertility regimen (or not undergoing removal of an ovary for medical reasons) be prohibited from donating eggs for research purposes only. This requirement that egg donors not be exposed to any incremental risk was probably stricter than was found in most NIH-funded research, in which normal volunteers often participate in risky studies. It reflected our belief that in the foreseeable future other donor sources would be available, that the risks outweighed any benefits, and that permitting healthy women to donate eggs for research could open the door to commercial exploitation. We did make one exception to this exclusion of women not involved in infertility procedures or not undergoing pelvic surgery. We permitted egg donation by such women when the aim was to establish a pregnancy. Our thinking was that this goal was sufficiently beneficial to permit—or at least not prohibit—healthy volunteers from exposing themselves to the added risks of stimulatory medications.

The report's fourth chapter also registered the outcome of one of our most heated discussions during the June meeting: the question of whether we would permit the use of eggs retrieved from deceased donors or fetuses. There was little doubt in anyone's mind that neither source was appropriate if the resulting embryo was to be transferred to a womb. The birth of a child whose biological mother was dead or had been aborted raised complex questions of lineage and identity for the child and others. But could these egg sources be used for otherwise acceptable research when transfer was not intended? We concluded that cadaver sources should be allowed if a woman had given permission for such research before she died, or if her relatives gave permission and she had not explicitly objected. This paralleled the regulations on organ donation.[211] In contrast, the use of fetal oocytes even with the permission of the woman undergoing abortion became such a source of controversy among us that we placed it in the category of research that "warrants additional review." Two considerations motivated this decision: the understanding that because fetal oocytes are very immature, they would be a poor source of eggs and the awareness that utilizing this source of eggs would unnecessarily implicate embryo research in the abortion and fetal tissue debates.

One final basic principle established in the report was an ethical distinction between the treatment of embryos intended for transfer (and birth) and those not intended for transfer. Embryos not intended for transfer, we agreed, could be exposed to potentially harmful interventions provided that researchers respected our other principles regarding minimum numbers and duration of research, donor consent, and the like. But we would prohibit the transfer of embryos that had been used in research "unless there is a reasonable confidence that any child born as a result of these procedures has not been harmed by them."[212] This would not rule out a level of risk already implicit in normal reproduction or in proven reproductive procedures. However, novel research—use of new growth media or innovative microsurgical procedures to enhance an embryo's chances of survival—could not be done unless there was solid reason to believe that they added no increased risk of birth defects. This distinction between embryos and children was at the very heart of our thinking. It reflected the scale of moral values that we had established and partly explained our support of embryo research, which was justified in terms of the health benefits to children and adults. The distinction also had to be plainly stated in our report, because those working in the field of reproductive medicine had not always respected it. They had often introduced new reproductive procedures without careful attention to the impact on the children born from them. Here was an instance in which federal funding could bring tighter control to the research enterprise.

The category "warrants additional review" occupied a good deal of our attention at the June meeting. Before dealing with this category, we had to decide what it meant. What kind of review did we (or the NIH) have in mind, and who would do the reviewing? Eventually, we would distinguish two very different types of additional review. One was an extra level of review for specific proposals that had been placed in the "acceptable" category but that needed further evaluation using sensitive ethical judgments. An example is the permission to create research embryos when doing so is "necessary for the validity of a study that is potentially of outstanding scientific and therapeutic value." If the NIH accepted this recommendation, someone would have to determine whether a study was sufficiently important to warrant the deliberate creation of research embryos. For this purpose, we recommended that the NIH form an ad hoc group that would continue to work for at least three years. This body would perform specific case-by-case evaluation of the kinds of "acceptable" research that required it. By building up knowledge and expertise in this area, it could serve as a source of information and education for IRBs during the initial years of embryo research. We assumed that local review boards would eventually assume this responsibility and that the ad hoc group would be phased out. Several years later, the NIH would propose a similar in-house group, the Human Pluripotent Stem Cell Review Group (HPSCRG), to oversee proposals for human stem cell research.[213]

We also made provision for the NIH to form another panel or group like ourselves in the future. This group might revisit any research directions that we now placed in the category of research that "warrants additional review." Our willingness to assign a number of research directions to this category reflected our belief that it is difficult to arrive at permanent prohibitions in an area in which the science is changing so rapidly. During our discussions it became clear that even some research in the "prohibited" category might have to be reconsidered eventually. Almost no prohibition can be absolute in a world in which today's imaginative possibility is tomorrow's widely demanded clinical procedure.

In authorizing both an ad hoc body and a future policy panel like ours, we were trying to avoid a repetition of the Ethics Advisory Board experience. History had shown that a congressionally mandated bioethics authority with the power to shut down whole areas of research is an invitation to purely political intervention in the research process. The ad hoc group we recommended was to be established at the discretion of the director of the NIH and could be phased out after three years. Any follow-up panel formed to reconsider research that we placed in the category "warrants additional review" would presumably come into being at the initiative of the NIH or other executive branch agencies. The aim was to maintain a degree of decentralization in oversight and to give the research community, supplemented by outside advisers, an important role in the ethical review process. Nothing in our experience suggested that researchers were unwilling to accept ethical oversight of their activities, provided that their input in the process was respected. A far greater risk than researcher dominance, we believed, was uninformed interventions by politicians responding to pressure group tactics.

Research placed in the category "warrants additional review" had two features: it was ethically controversial and its feasibility or benefit was not yet established. It made sense, then, to wait until the picture cleared. The final report assigned five items to this category: (1) cloning by blastomere separation or blastocyst splitting, without transfer; (2) research performed between the appearance of the primitive streak and the beginning of closure of the neural tube; (3) research that uses fetal oocytes for fertilization, without transfer, or for parthenogenesis; (4) nuclear transplantation into an enucleated, fertilized, or unfertilized (but activated) egg, with transfer, for the purpose of circumventing or correcting an inherited cytoplasmic defect; and (5) embryonic stem cell research that uses deliberately fertilized oocytes.

The fourth and fifth items on the list illustrate the concerns that motivated us to assign items to this category. The fourth item, therapeutic nuclear transfer, is controversial because it involves techniques that can also be used in somatic cell nuclear transfer (SCNT) cloning and the creation of one or more genetic copies of a living individual. Worries about the broader implications of cloning would arise a few years down the line following the cloning of the sheep Dolly. In this case, however, the goal is not to clone a particular individual, but to provide therapy for a serious genetic disorder. A growing number of conditions are being traced to mutations in the mitichondria, small RNA-bearing bodies that control energy use and that are transmitted to the embryo through the egg's cytoplasm. Every child born to a woman whose eggs are affected in this way will inherit the diseased RNA. Clinicians seeking to help someone with this problem can extract the nucleus from an embryo created with one of her eggs and transfer it to a "healthy" donor egg the nucleus of which has been removed. Because the nucleus carries the overwhelming amount of genetic material, the child will be very much like any other child of the woman—but free of the mitochondrial disorder. Much work remains before this technology can be used reliably to produce healthy children. Among other things, it remains to be seen whether a nucleus can be sufficiently cleansed of any residual maternal cytoplasm to assure the birth of a child free of the mitochondrial disease. Because of the sensitivity of this research and the need for much preliminary animal work on the safety of cloning procedures, we decided to let another review body look at this issue a few years later.[214]

Similar reasoning applied to the fifth item on this list: embryonic stem cell (ES) research. In the course of our discussions, we learned that this is an area of enormous promise. Brigid Hogan regarded ES research as one of the most important topics we would consider. Her laboratory at Vanderbilt had pioneered mouse research in this area, and she believed that research on human stem cells was imminent. Brigid agreed that, in the foreseeable future, spare embryos would suffice for the development of the basic techniques that would be needed. This research went into our "acceptable" category. But what about the use of embryos deliberately created for this purpose? We were ready to approve the use of research embryos when fertilization was a necessary end point of the research and when research was needed for studies of outstanding scientific and therapeutic value. Neither of these categories seemed to apply to the initial phases of human stem cell research, for which spare embryos would suffice.

Brigid's gaze, however, was set on a slightly more distant future. She knew that if human ES cell lines could be developed and proved to be of therapeutic value, a clinical need would soon arise for diverse immunologically compatible cell lines suitable for different ethnic groups and classes of individuals. It was unlikely that these lines would be produced from existing spare embryos. Hence the need for deliberately created embryos. What were we to say now about an activity that might become very important in the future? Carol Tauer believed that this possibility should be placed in the "unacceptable" category. She argued that the production of therapeutic cell lines did not have to involve federally funded research but was a matter for private tissue banks and distribution networks. Other panel members were not convinced these capabilities could be developed without extensive prior research. Nevertheless, reasoning that the need for research in this area was not imminent, we placed it in the category "warrants additional review." Carol Tauer took issue with this conclusion to write one of the report's few dissents.[215]

Our debates about these issues became a useful matter of record. In 1998 the Geron Corporation organized its own ethics advisory board to assist with oversight of its funding of stem cell research. The recommendations of that board drew on our panel's work. Although our recommendations had no immediate impact at the federal level, they did prove influential in helping direct the course of private research. As it turned out, our decision to permit some aspects of this research, such as the use of spare embryos for this purpose, corresponded fairly well to the emerging state of science. This is testimony to the value of having had a cutting-edge scientist like Brigid Hogan in our midst.

This same pair of considerations—ethical uncertainty and uncertain benefits—applied to the four other items we classified as "warrants additional review." Evidence indicated that item 1, J. L. Hall's work on cloning by blastomere separation, would not be an effective way of multiplying the number of viable embryos available to couples.[216] Although technological breakthroughs might alter this situation in the future,[217] the many controversial ethical questions raised by induced twinning recommended against our approving it then. Item 2, the prospect of *in vitro* research on embryos between the appearance of the primitive streak and the beginning of the closure of the neural tube, remained science fiction. It was barely possible to keep embryos alive and intact *in vitro* for more than a few days after fertilization. We heard arguments about the possible importance for neuroscience of research during this brief interval when the nervous system begins to form and when so many genes are uniquely expressed, but it hardly seemed necessary at this time to challenge the international consensus that drew a line at the formation of the primitive streak. Item 3, the matter of using fetal oocytes, was easily dismissed. Brigid Hogan drew our attention to the fact that fetal oocytes might someday be useful as a source of research embryos or parthenotes in studies in which a control group was needed that had not been exposed to environmental toxins, but it was unlikely that very immature eggs of this sort could be used in the near future. This did not support our wading into the complex issue of using fetal eggs as a source.

The third and final category, "unacceptable research," was the one to which we gave the least thought. This was partly because of the fatigue and time pressure that overwhelmed us in the final hours of our June meeting. In addition, some of the proposed research in this category was so obviously questionable both in scientific and ethical terms that it certainly would not merit federal support in the foreseeable future. In the final report, we identified four ethical considerations that led us to place research in this category. They included the potentially adverse consequences of the research for children, women, and men; the respect due the preimplantation embryo; concern for public sensitivities about highly controversial research proposals; and concern for the meaning of humanness, parenthood, and the succession of generations. We also concluded that all the items placed in this category were of very minor scientific or therapeutic value.

The final report included ten items in this category: (1) cloning of human preimplantation embryos by separating blastomeres or dividing blastocysts (induced twinning), followed by transfer to a womb; (2) studies designed to transplant nuclei into an enucleated egg, including nuclear cloning, in order to duplicate a genome or to increase the number of embryos with the same genotype, with transfer; (3) research beyond the onset of closure of the neural tube; (4) research involving the fertilization of fetal oocytes with transfer; (5) preimplantation genetic diagnosis for sex selection except to avoid the transmission of sex-linked genetic diseases; (6) development of human–nonhuman and human–human chimeras with or without transfer; (7) cross-species fertilization except to conduct clinical tests of the ability of sperm to penetrate eggs; (8) attempted transfer of parthenogenetically activated human eggs; (9) attempted transfer of human embryos into nonhuman animals for gestation; and (10) transfer of human embryos for the induction of extra-uterine or abdominal pregnancy.

Despite the lack of full discussion and debate about all the items on this list, their inclusion in the category of unacceptable research seemed reasonable. Sometimes the matter was open-and-shut. Even if it could be done, cross-species fertilization (item 7) poses massive risks for any children born as a result of such manipulations. Even now, in the wake of Dolly, cloning research the aim of which is to produce a live birth (item 2) is far too risky for the child and raises many other unresolved ethical questions. It is pointless and possibly hazardous to transfer a parthenote to a woman's womb (item 8), because it cannot possibly continue to develop normally. Other items on this list were arguably of greater value. We heard an argument, for example, that the creation of human-human chimeras, the deliberate mixing of cell lines from different embryos (item 6), may be one future route to gene therapy. For example, because of a genetic mutation, the cells of an individual suffering from cystic fibrosis fail to produce a structure essential to salt transport. The result is the destructive accumulation of mucus throughout the body, especially in the lungs. In the future, it might be possible to correct these problems by seeding an embryo with one or more healthy cells. But clearly the science is underdeveloped and, where transfer is involved, the risks for born children are unknown. Someday, too, a technology of inducing extrauterine pregnancies (item 10) will be developed to help women who lack a uterus to have a child. Such pregnancies sometimes occur spontaneously when an egg leaves the fallopian tube and lodges outside the womb, but this can be life threatening. Unlike some of the other items on this list, research in this area is not pointless. But to some members of the public, the prospect of inducing extrauterine pregnancies invokes visions of men having children. We did not wish to stir up these fears. True, there were research directions that stimulated public apprehensions for which we were willing to recommend funding. Parthenogenesis research without transfer is a good example. But these areas had important scientific and therapeutic value and, thus, we were willing to defend them in the face of purely emotional reactions. In contrast, we found no compelling reasons to support any item on the list of unacceptable research.

As far as embryo research was concerned, the summer was deceptively quiet. The topic had almost vanished from the newspapers and science journals. Preparing for a late September rollout of our completed report, the NIH was readying press packets that explained the science of embryo research and outlined our recommendations. Several independent scientists and ethicists were enlisted to explain these materials in a special briefing planned for the press. As Kathi Hanna finished the task of converting our draft chapters into a final report, NIH staff used e-mail and fax to re-poll us on some close or ambiguous votes. We had every reason to believe our report would be well received and that most of our recommendations would soon go into effect.

On 27 September, with the report bound and ready for distribution, most members of the panel reassembled in Washington for the official announcement of our recommendations. We gathered in a large meeting room at the NIH. In addition to NIH administrators and scientists, several dozen representatives of the national press and camera crews from the major networks were present. Several panel members had been asked to offer summaries of the parts of the report for which they were responsible. After Brigid introduced the science issues, I followed with a brief presentation of our thinking on the moral status of the preimplantation embryo. I stressed the need to approach the issue from the perspective of acceptable public policy in a society in which many views compete. Americans, I said, hold "very different views on the question of the moral value of prenatal life at its various stages." The aim of a panel like ours was not to decide which of these views is right, but rather to arrive at a "reasonable accommodation to diverse interests." Our recommendations, which permitted embryo research under strict constraints, tried to do just that. I closed by outlining the reasons we were willing to permit the deliberate fertilization of eggs—research embryos—for selected purposes.

In the questioning that followed, a reporter immediately asked, "Where does the soul fit into all this?" I replied by saying that this was a spiritual question that individuals and religious faiths might address, but not something that a public panel like ours could answer. As I spoke, I realized how unsatisfactory this reply must be to millions of people who believed— hoped?—that a collection of ethicists and scientists could somehow pinpoint the appearance of the soul. This hope was unreasonable, but its persistence indicated the formidable obstacles facing any recommendations for public support of embryo research.

Although the September event went well, the controversy was just beginning. Journalist Eliot Marshall, writing in *Science,* predicted that the NIH faced "a sizzling autumn" as a result of our report.[218] Right-to-life organizations kept up their drumbeat of opposition. This was expected, but opposition from those who normally supported reproductive medicine and abortion rights was not. Dissenters focused principally on our recommendation regarding the creation of research embryos. Arthur Caplan, perhaps the country's best known "public bioethicist," wrote a syndicated newspaper column in which he dismissed this recommendation, terming it a proposal for "designer embryos." Caplan's choice of terminology confused embryo research with public fears about genetic manipulations and did not advance reasoned debate.

Unfortunately for our work, Caplan was not alone in his opposition to this recommendation. An unsigned lead editorial in the Sunday, 2 October edition of the *Washington Post* indicated that, despite strong support for this recommendation among panel members, it was not going to win public acceptance. The editorial praised our work as "a conscientious effort to answer a question fraught with difficulties both moral and scientific" and described most of our recommendations as "useful." However, it called our recommendation regarding research embryos "flat wrong" and "unconscionable." One did not have to be against abortion rights or believe that human life begins at conception, the editorial continued, "to be deeply alarmed by the notion of scientists' purposely causing conceptions in a context entirely divorced from even the potential of reproduction." No argument was given as to why it was morally acceptable to produce excess embryos for reproductive purposes, embryos almost certain to be destroyed, but not permissible to do so for vital health-related research. Clearly, arguments were not in order. It was enough to invoke the image of scientists creating life in the laboratory to show that it should not be done. The editorial closed by taking note of Pat King's dissent from the second of the two conditions under which we would permit the creation of research embryos, but disagreed with even her qualified permission. Any government funding for research embryos, it said, is "a step too far."

The storm clouds thickened appreciably after the November election. Although Newt Gingrich's "contract with America" dealt largely with economic issues, the new Republican majority brought with it the return of a conservative social agenda that included opposition to abortion and to advances in reproductive medicine, an agenda that had prevailed during two previous Republican administrations. It would be months before it became clear what forms this conservative policy might take, but there was no reason to believe that any NIH funding of human embryo research would be exempt from attack.

One could almost feel the atmosphere of gloom as the Advisory Committee to the Director (ACD) of the NIH met on 2 December in the same conference room in which our report had been aired in more optimistic circumstances a few months before. As ACD members debated the report, phrases like "the need to be realistic" and "political repercussions" floated about. Nan Keohane, who was a member both of our panel and the ACD, spoke forcefully about the value of this research and described the process that led to our recommendations. Harold Varmus added his voice to Nan's and praised the panel's recommendations. Later, there were reports that at just this moment Varmus was under pressure from the White House to trim our recommendations in order to avoid the need for presidential involvement. However, he evidenced none of this pressure in his remarks. He displayed a little-noted "profile in courage" in defense of the integrity of the science policy review process.

Varmus's leadership had its expected effect. Despite the gloomy atmosphere, by midday the ACD voted unanimously to accept our recommendations. This was the formal step needed to authorize NIH funding of human embryo research. In the weeks ahead, NIH administrators and lawyers would convert our recommendations into draft regulatory guidelines that could be published for a sixty-day period of public review. When this period ended, perhaps within a few months, research proposals already in the NIH pipeline could be funded.

Later that afternoon I treated myself to a glass of wine on the plane as I returned to Hanover. The ACD's substantial vote of support suggested that our recommendations might actually see the light of day. Arriving home, I had barely taken off my coat when my wife, Mary Jean, handed me the phone. On the line was a reporter from *The New York Times* asking for my response to the president's action. "What action?" I asked in puzzlement. The reporter then read to me a brief statement by President Clinton released by the White House after our meeting had ended. In it he expressed appreciation for the work of our panel and agreed that "advances in *in vitro* fertilization research and other areas could derive from such work." He then added, "However, I do not believe that federal funds should be used to support the creation of human embryos for research purposes, and I have directed that NIH not allocate any resources for such research." The statement closed by noting that "in order to insure that advice on complex bioethical issues that affect our society can continue to be developed, we are planning to move forward with the establishment of a National Bioethics Advisory Commission over the next year."[219]

I told the reporter that I was surprised that members of the panel had never been told of the administration's views and added that I did not want to comment beyond that. I recall the sense of anger and betrayal I felt as I hung up the phone, even though a rejection of this recommendation was reasonable. This was probably the best way to salvage the possibility that some initial embryo research could go forward, using parthenotes or the spare embryos that were available. When I calmed down a few days later, I told friends there might be some political logic to the president's move. By sacrificing our most controversial recommendation, he may have hoped to appease the report's most vociferous critics. However, if this was the White House's intent, it did not achieve its purpose. This capitulation may have even bolstered the opposition to NIH funding in this area. Whatever the wisdom of one political strategy or another, it was rankling that the White House had intervened in this manner. Administration spokesmen had had months to communicate their views on this issue. Abruptly overruling our recommendations without prior warning sent the message that a policy panel was, at best, an ornament that could be used or discarded as political needs demanded. Over the next few years, this approach by Clinton's science policy staff would evidence itself in other forms.[220]

A year later I attended a conference of the Association for Practical and Professional Ethics, where the keynote speaker was William A. Galston, White House deputy assistant for domestic policy. Galston's address reviewed his role in forming the president's position on embryo research and in preparing the 2 December statement. He spoke at length on the political forces that were bearing down on the White House at that time and reported that the *Washington Post*'s October editorial was a major negative factor in the administration's thinking. Galston continued by developing a long moral argument against the creation of research embryos, focusing on "slippery slopes" and the possible instrumentalization of human life. He made no mention at all of any arguments on the other side of the issue or the reasons why our panel had come to a different conclusion.

After simmering for an hour, I spoke up during the question and answer session that followed. I explained that, as a member of the panel, I wanted to point out that we had arrived at our recommendations for good reasons. These included the ongoing risks in current clinical activities that might be reduced by use of research embryos. I concluded by mentioning a "slippery slope" that Galston failed to consider. In the area of reproductive medicine, I said, independent panels had repeatedly seen their work ignored or over-turned by administration or congressional action. Witness, I urged, the fate of the 1979 Ethics Advisory Board report[221] and that of the Fetal Tissue Trans-plantation Panel in the late 1980s.[222] "What is the impact on qualified people's willingness to serve on these panels and do this work," I asked, "if their recommendations are routinely ignored? And what happens to public policy in a field like reproductive medicine when abrupt political decisions are al-lowed to override months of thoughtful study and debate?"[223] Galston replied that the White House's decision had not been precipitous, that "weeks and months of thinking" had preceded it. I knew that we were not going to con-vince one another, but I was pleased to have had the chance to alert others to the issues and, frankly, to voice this grievance.

The highly politicized nature of these debates was driven home to me once more before the end of 1994. Late in December I received a call from the NIH Office of Science Policy with a request. PBS's *McNeil-Lehrer News Hour* wished to air a debate between a panel spokesperson and Bernadine Healy on the matter of embryo research. Steven Muller had declined this role, and Pat King was unavailable. "Would you represent the panel?" I agreed to do so and flew to New York for that night's show. I would be facing Robin McNeil in the New York studio; Healy would be off-site in Akron, Ohio.

Bernadine Healy had served as director of the NIH during the latter part of the Bush administration. In that role, she had made some very important contributions to furthering health-related research for women, but her record of support for reproductive research was not good. She had done nothing, for example, to implement the Fetal Tissue Transplantation Research Panel's rec-ommendations.[224] During the preceding year, she had run, unsuccessfully, as a Republican candidate for the Senate from Ohio. I suspect she saw this debate as a chance to firm up her "pro-life" credentials among conservative voters.

The debate itself, which occupied ten minutes of airtime, was an exhilarat-ing experience. I was well enough steeped in the issues to respond sensibly, I thought, to Robin McNeil's sharp questions. Healy took a position rejecting all embryo research on the grounds that it violated the rights of tiny human subjects. In general, she did not come across as particularly knowledgeable about the issues, and McNeil had to repeat some questions to her without getting a clear answer. As the debate drew to a close, I felt that I was able to convey the seriousness of the reasoning behind our panel's recommendations. I also hoped that I had made this a less successful political foray than Healy had intended. At the close of the show, a staff member led me through the maze of studio corridors to the elevator. I knew I had not let the panel down when the elevator door opened and I faced a crowd of PBS staff, mostly women. Recognizing me from the just-completed broadcast, they broke into applause.

Unfortunately, female voters living and working on the Upper West Side of Manhattan do not determine U.S. reproductive policy. Within a matter of months, the dramatic changes that had been ushered in by the Clinton administration were reversed as the newly conservative congress finally addressed the issue. In August 1995 representatives Jay Dickey (R-Ark.) and Roger Wicker (R-Miss.) offered an amendment to a vote by the House Appropriations Committee that would bar researchers who receive funds from the Department of Health and Human Services (which includes the NIH) from using human embryos created by private *in vitro* fertilization services. The amendment was passed into law in January 1996.[225] An effort later that year by John Porter (R-IL.), the Labor Appropriations Subcommittee chair and an NIH supporter, to replace it in the next year's funding bill with a less comprehensive amendment that would permit some use of spare embryos was defeated.[226] That vote followed a committee action that banned the funding of most abortions by the federal employees' health insurance program, the government's principal family planning program. The *Washington Post* reported that all of these items were high on the legislative agenda of the Christian Coalition, which had been stepping up pressure on Republicans to finally deliver results. "We're taking this one step at a time," said Rep. Christopher H. Smith (R-N.J.), a leader of the anti-abortion forces. "We're not going to underwrite the killing of unborn children."[227]

Thus, the work of our panel concluded with the onset of a new "ice age" for federally funded human embryo research. The next few years would see dramatic developments in the private sector and overseas, not the least of which was the November 1998 announcement of the development of human stem cell lines. Not until this and other private sector activities forged ahead did the issue of embryo research surface. Then, the fear that somehow the government had lost its ability to oversee this novel research and that the private sector would reap all the benefits of whatever research was done reawakened a sleeping public and Congress.

6

THE CLONING
CONTROVERSY

O NE result of my year of service on the Embryo Research Panel was a lingering case of "Beltway fever," a desire to be near the center of public policy formation in bioethics. I had long been susceptible to this affliction. My work in bioethics had always focused on public ethical choices, such as questions of social justice in population policy, reproductive medicine, and health care access.[228] As an ethicist, I believed that clear and rigorous thinking about difficult new issues could help make a difference in the way a society responded to them. The Human Embryo Research Panel was a chance to apply this belief.

Late in 1995 I was given another opportunity to do so when I was approached with a job offer by Jeffrey Trent, scientific director of the Division of Intramural Research at the NIH's National Center for Human Genome Research (NCHGR). The NCHGR—later to be upgraded to the status of a full NIH institute and renamed the National Human Genome Research Institute (NHGRI)—is the main federal funding and research center for the Human Genome Project, the massive, ten-year-long effort to identify and sequence the estimated three billion base pair chemical units that make up the human genetic code, or genome.[229] Most NCHGR/NHGRI resources go to an extramural research program that supports genetic research at universities and research institutions around the world. In 1989, at the urging of James D.

Watson, the codiscoverer of DNA and then head of the center, NCHGR established an extramural research program in the "Ethical, Legal and Social Implications" (ELSI) of the human genome project. Although only about five percent of NCHGR's total resources are devoted to this program, it nevertheless represents an unprecedented commitment to anticipatory research on a branch of science whose impact on society is potentially enormous.

Like most other NIH institutes, NCHGR/NHGRI also maintains an intramural research program on the NIH campus in Bethesda, Md. Here, a group of several hundred professionals in the fields of microbiology, medical genetics, and genetic counseling work to identify the genes involved in various disorders and to explore the applications of this knowledge to clinical care. Jeff explained to me that those researchers frequently confront unfamiliar ethical questions in the course of their research and clinical efforts. The ELSI program addressed some of these questions, but its scholarly findings were not readily usable by busy intramural researchers. They needed somebody on-site to assist them. Jeff had come to know me in the course of some consulting work I had done for the NIH's program in clinical bioethics. Over a lunch in Washington in late 1995, he asked whether I would be willing to come to Bethesda—part-time, full-time, for a shorter or longer period—to help set up an office of "genome ethics" in the intramural division.

The offer came at a good time. I welcomed the chance to learn from researchers at the forefront of genetic research, and I hoped that I could make a contribution to furthering their understanding of its ethical implications. On the personal front, I was free for the first time in my life to be away from home for extended periods. Our two children were off to college and graduate school, and my wife had just been appointed dean of humanities at Dartmouth. With several years of faculty dinners and department retreats ahead of her, she was willing to let me spend part of my time in Washington.

In January 1996, right in the midst of Newt Gingrich's shutdown of the federal government, I started my work at NCHGR. For the next eighteen months I commuted on a week-on, week-off basis between Bethesda and Hanover. The challenge was enormous. I had to administer a small staff with some fixed responsibilities, including the development of a basic course on scientific research ethics for all genome center researchers, while also trying to define the role of an "office of genome ethics" in a large genetic research program. The learning curve was steep. There was a need to familiarize myself with basic microbiology and medical genetics. Novel bioethical questions presented themselves every day.

A large part of my time was devoted to issues of informed consent. The unique feature of genetic research is the predominantly "social" nature of genetic information. It is one thing for people to consent to participate in research aimed at discovering genes involved in cancer or other serious disorders, but what does it mean when that consent affects others who share those same genes? For example, I might be willing to donate a blood sample for prostate cancer research, and, in so doing, I might even be willing to accept the risks of future genetic discrimination in employment or insurance. But is it permissible to subject my children to this risk? The problem extends beyond families. Some disease conditions run in ethnic or racial groups. For example, among Jews of eastern European (Ashkenazic) background, particular mutations of the BRCA1 and BRCA2 genes seem to be associated with a higher incidence of breast and ovarian cancer in women and prostate cancer in men. Some people of Native American background share genes that may predispose them to alcoholism. Will an individual's or family's participation in research on these genes foster discrimination for all members of the group?[230]

By June 1997 the burden of commuting weekly between Washington and Hanover and the toll of trying to do two full-time jobs had grown fairly heavy. I had accomplished my task of helping to identify and implement some of the key functions of the office. A committee of scientists and administrators reviewed our work and committed the institute to continuing the office under a full-time director. My "Beltway fever" had run its course. Although I looked forward to occasional trips to Washington and Bethesda to assist with thinking and research on substantive ethical issues, I was eager to return to the opportunities for teaching, research, and writing afforded by a more private academic life.

It was probably good that in the several years following the work of the Human Embryo Research Panel my mind was on matters other than embryo research. In terms of federal support for such research, this was a bleak period. The first Republican congress since 1954 was vigorously pursuing its "Contract with America." Most public attention was focused on economic issues, but conservative Republican and Democratic members of Congress also had social objectives. Foremost among them were efforts to reverse the Clinton administration's initiatives in abortion policy and reproductive medicine.

When it finally passed into law in January 1996, the Dickey-Wicker amendment to the annual appropriations bill for the Department of Health and Human Services ended the possibility of federally funded embryo research. The amendment prohibited funding for "the creation of a human embryo or embryos for research purposes" as well as "research in which a human embryo or embryos are destroyed, discarded, or knowingly subjected to risk of injury or death greater than that allowed for research on fetuses in utero" under existing federal regulations.[231] Existing fetal regulations permit researchers to impose risks on a fetus that are needed to meet its "health needs." In the case of research activities that confer no direct medical benefit on the fetus, the regulations permit only "minimal" risks.[232] This is a slightly more stringent standard than applies to pediatric research, where greater than minimal risks are allowed when the research is likely to yield "knowledge . . . of vital importance for the understanding or amelioration of the subjects' disorder or condition."[233] Children, in other words, can be involved in research, with their parents' or guardians' consent, even when the research is somewhat risky and does not benefit them, if it can produce knowledge of more general value related to their disorder. Thanks to the Dickey-Wicker amendment, the preimplantation embryo, like the fetus before it, was now regarded in U.S. law as being even more protectable than a child.

Dickey-Wicker also revealed that the Human Embryo Research Panel's extended debates about spare versus research embryos were irrelevant. The new conservative congress would permit almost *no* embryo research. It made no difference whether the embryos were deliberately created for research or left over from infertility procedures and destined to be discarded. Despite the expectations of my panel colleagues, even parthenogenesis research for medical benefit would now, for the first time, be explicitly denied federal support. Parthenotes are not embryos and cannot possibly develop beyond a few cleavage stages. But the amendment defined "the human embryo or embryos" as "any organism . . . that is derived by fertilization, parthenogenesis, cloning, or any other means from one or more human gametes or diploid cells."

As dismal as this picture was, Dickey-Wicker could have been worse. As an amendment to a federal appropriations bill, it had to be renewed annually. Furthermore, its prohibitions did not cover privately funded research. Whereas in Britain regulations developed by the Human Fertilisation and Embryology Authority (HFEA) govern all embryo research conducted in that country, in this country the activities of private clinics would not be directly affected by the Dickey-Wicker ban. Nevertheless, until the makeup of Congress changed or the negative implications of this ban became more apparent to the public, there would be no federal support for embryo research or areas of reproductive medicine that depend on it.[234]

Despite legislators' efforts, science does not stand still. One way or another, scientists will pursue enticing research possibilities, driven by their understanding of where the most important questions lie and where answers may be found. Almost predictably, the event that reopened the debate about embryo research took place beyond the reach of the U.S. Congress. In the summer of 1996, as the result of work by an obscure team of researchers at Scotland's Roslin Institute, Dolly, the first mammal ever produced by somatic cell nuclear transfer cloning technology, was born. The Roslin team, led by Ian Wilmut and Keith Campbell, inserted the nucleus of a cell taken from one sheep's udder into another sheep's egg, the nucleus of which had been removed by microsurgery. They then applied an electric current to stimulate the new diploid cell to start dividing and transferred the resulting embryo to a third sheep's womb. Dolly's birth was kept secret for months while the Roslin researchers verified what they had done and prepared a scientific report. This was published in the February 1997 issue of *Nature*.[235]

The experiment leading to Dolly was not directly related to human reproduction. HFEA regulations explicitly prohibit human cloning. In cloning Dolly, the Roslin researchers (and their financial backers at PPL Therapeutics, Ltd.) were trying to produce a genetically uniform line of farm animals that might be useful in the future as living "factories" for pharmaceutical products.[236] Nevertheless, the implications of Dolly for human reproduction were clear. Press accounts and commentators quickly asked how long it would be before human cloning took place.

Future historians of science and culture who look back on the debates and actions that followed the announcement of Dolly will find rich material for comment and reflection. In one respect, the public underestimated the truly revolutionary impact of the Roslin team's work.[237] A remarkable feature of biology is that every cell in a multicellular organism contains the genetic program for the organism as a whole. It is as though every brick and girder in a huge skyscraper were to contain the complete blueprint—and construction crew—for the entire building. However, once a living organism moves beyond the earliest embryonic stages, this genetic blueprint becomes largely inoperative and inaccessible. Most of it is filed away, and only a very small subset of genetic instructions needed for each cell's specialized work is used. What Wilmut and Campbell discovered was a means of reopening and reactivating those closed files. They did this by starving the cell's nucleus into a quiescent state and inserting it into an enucleated egg. This somehow permitted material in the egg's cytoplasm to reactivate the whole repertoire of nuclear genes. Implicit in their work was a vast new field of biological control and medical interventions. The production of specialized cells, tissues, or even organs-to-order for animal or human uses was now possible.

But these possible benefits were not what fascinated the public. It was the threat of human cloning that drew attention and that was frequently overestimated. Some of the nightmare visions bothering the public were barely rooted in scientific reality. In the public imagination, cloned armies of superwarriors marched at the command of new biological tyrants, despite the fact that any dictator choosing this path to domination would have to wait at least two decades for his cloned army to grow up. Writers wondered whether clones would have souls, ignoring the fact that millions of natural clones— identical twins—already live among us.

To some extent, of course, these overreactions were understandable. Generations of novels and movies—from *Brave New World* to *The Boys from Brazil* to *Multiplicity*—had conditioned the public to see cloning as a threat to human freedom and individuality. It is not surprising that within hours or days of Dolly's announcement, negative reactions predominated. Religious leaders from all sides of the spectrum of theological opinion hastened to declare human cloning ethically unacceptable.[238] Around the world governments and international organizations raced to impose bans on cloning research.[239] In the United States, President Clinton used his executive powers to institute a moratorium on any federal research leading to the cloning of a human being. He also asked his newly appointed National Bioethics Advisory Commission (NBAC) to study the issue and report back to him within ninety days with recommendations on possible federal actions to prevent the abuse of cloning.[240]

One side effect of Dolly's birth was renewed attention to human embryo research. If human cloning were ever to be accomplished, it would be necessary to apply the techniques developed for Dolly to human embryos. This meant that many experimental cloned human embryos would have to be created before the first birth of a cloned child would even be possible. This reappearance of the issue of embryo research in the context of the cloning debate was unfortunate. It reinforced opposition to embryo research generally and strengthened the hand of those who would use the law to prohibit any research in this area. Not surprisingly, in the wake of Dolly's announcement, new proposals were aired in Congress to extend the ban on federal funding to include a ban on privately funded human embryo research as well.[241]

These efforts at prohibition were unlikely to succeed, but they also ensured that whatever cloning research eventually took place would proceed without federal oversight. Within weeks of the announcement of Dolly's birth, reports began to circulate that for-profit companies—at least one of which identified itself as being located in the Cayman Islands—were racing to develop and offer cloning as a reproductive option. These reports were either spurious, or, as in the case of the Chicago physicist Richard Seed, who announced his intention to clone a child,[242] reflected wishful thinking rather than scientific capability. Nevertheless, the reports pointed to a larger lesson. Neither the federal government's refusal to support this research area nor even an outright legal ban on it would stop human embryo or cloning research. This research would continue covertly in this country or in overseas laboratories not reached by U.S. laws. By a kind of scientific Gresham's law, these efforts at prohibition would only increase the chances that the most unregulated and irresponsible research would prevail.

Amid this turmoil, the president's new NBAC began its work. It met for the first time in October 1996. Producing a report on cloning was its first responsibility. In some respects, NBAC was a different kind of group than the Human Embryo Research Panel. The White House brought it into being, mandating that it provide advice to executive branch agencies on a range of bioethics issues, including human subjects protections. Its life span was indeterminate. Although the initial term of service was set at two years and was later extended by two years, there was reason to believe it would continue to exist as long as it continued to perform useful service. In contrast, the embryo panel had been formed by one executive branch agency, the NIH, to provide guidance on a specific issue, and it went out of existence with the completion of its task. NBAC's members were presidentially appointed commissioners, whereas the embryo panel's members were temporary consultants. Despite these differences, however, there were some interesting similarities between the two groups. Most striking, perhaps, was some continuity in membership. Three of NBAC's seventeen commissioners, Alta Charo, Tom Murray, and Bernard Lo, had also served on the embryo panel. Like the embryo panel, NBAC was a multidisciplinary group, with research scientists, physicians, ethicists, lawyers, and policy analysts among its members. Like the embryo panel, NBAC was an executive branch entity. This meant that its recommendations would eventually go before a conservative—and largely hostile—Congress. Finally, the assignment of a report on cloning to NBAC meant that, once again, after a pause of barely two years, a federal expert panel was trying to come up with advice and guidelines in a controversial area of reproductive medicine. The ongoing human embryo research debates were being renewed.

NBAC performed as asked. In June 1997, just two weeks behind schedule, it published its report, *Cloning Human Beings*.[243] The report noted the complexity of the ethical issues raised by cloning. Many of those who testified during commission hearings expressed concerns about the harms that cloning might cause.[244] Among them was psychological damage to the resulting children, including a possibly diminished sense of individuality and personal autonomy.[245] Others expressed concern about a degradation in the quality of parenting and family life.[246] Some feared that cloning would open the door to new forms of eugenics.[247]

In its report, NBAC chose to mute these broader concerns and focus its attention on the specific physiological risks for any children brought into being by cloning. The Roslin team had constructed 277 embryos from the mammary cells of a Finn-Dorset sheep. Of these, only 29 showed enough development to permit their transfer to the wombs of surrogate mothers. All but one of these transferred embryos either failed to implant or stopped developing *in utero*.[248] It also was not clear that Dolly, the survivor, was in perfect physical health. Among the fears were that she might have inherited harmful mutations or premature aging from the somatic cell used to create her.[249] For these reasons, the NBAC report concluded that at this time human cloning "would be a premature experiment that would expose the fetus and the developing child to unacceptable risks."[250]

On this basis, NBAC recommended continuation of the moratorium that President Clinton had imposed on federal funding for any attempts to create a child in this way. It also asked for immediate voluntary compliance with this research moratorium in the private sector. Finally, it called for federal legislation to prohibit anyone from attempting, whether in a research or clinical setting, to create a child through somatic cell nuclear transfer cloning. Such legislation, the report added, should include a "sunset" provision requiring Congress to review the issue after a specified time period (three to five years) in order to decide whether the prohibition would continue to be needed.[251]

In some respects, the NBAC report is a judicious document. Although criticized by some for not giving more attention to the social and psychological concerns many people have raised about cloning, NBAC was wise to ground its recommendations on the most immediate risks. Also positive was NBAC's careful effort to distinguish attempts to clone a human being from cloning research generally. Only the effort to clone a child threatens imminent harms. In contrast, cloning, whether with animals or, eventually, with human embryos not intended for transfer to a womb, was a key new research technique for understanding cellular differentiation and embryological development. Banning it would shut down a promising area of biomedical research. Finally, the recommendation for a sunset clause was a laudable attempt to avoid creating a permanent obstacle to progress. As we learned so well on the Human Embryo Research Panel, life sciences research is moving so fast that today's troubling science fiction fantasies often become tomorrow's clinical applications. No prohibitions should be immune to review.

Despite all this, I believe that NBAC's handling of the cloning issue was seriously deficient. In fact, I regard it as a case study in poorly conducted public bioethics. This is true both of the way that NBAC responded to the president's request—its process—as well as the substance of the commission's final report. In several important respects, it provides an unfortunate model for public policy making in the area of reproductive science. In what follows, I will develop these criticisms of NBAC and draw some comparisons with the Human Embryo Research Panel. I do so for two reasons. First, NBAC's handling of the cloning issue contributed to the neglect of human embryo research in U.S. public policy. It is thus another chapter in the long history of neglect that marks this area. Second, the failure to address the issue of embryo research soon became glaring when the issue of stem cells arose not long afterward. In the next chapter I will show how the patterns that NBAC established in its considerations of cloning also marred its approach to the stem cell issue and clouded public discussion of a matter far more important than cloning itself.

Obviously, my criticisms should be viewed with caution. First, I have an investment in the way that the Embryo Panel approached its job of addressing a very controversial issue in reproductive medicine. NBAC diverged from the panel's approach on several matters; my partisanship here is unavoidable.

I also acknowledge that NBAC worked under difficult conditions. Newly created and operating with a partial staff and uncertain budget, NBAC's members were asked by President Clinton to produce a report on a very complex bioethical issue in just ninety days. That NBAC completed the report is an achievement. Nevertheless, problems with the report and process are worth highlighting because they continue to some extent into the present and are also evident in the later stem cell report. As such, they represent an unfortunate pattern that continues to perturb policy making about reproductive research in this country.

The problematic pattern began when NBAC ceded to the president's request to produce a report in three months. My first criticism is that NBAC even chose to accept this assignment. At the outset, NBAC's members made a strategic decision that they would try, in such a short time, to provide advice on an issue of enormous complexity the scientific and technical dimensions of which were still far from clear. Political scientist Andrea Bonnicksen asked a fair question: "What was the rush?"[252] No one reasonably believed that the announcement of Dolly would soon lead to efforts to clone a human being. Why accept this hurried time frame? From my experience on the embryo panel, I understand that national commissions have a built-in tendency to try to please those who create them.[253] NBAC was formed at the president's urging, and it is always difficult to turn down a presidential request. I also understand that with a designated two-year term of service, NBAC's members felt they had little time to waste. Nevertheless, NBAC might have considered whether it first should have asked for more time for study and deliberation. A time frame of one year to produce a report on the issue or the opportunity to periodically reexamine it while continuing to monitor and report on developments would not have been unreasonable. As I will try to show, this rush to judgment flaws the argumentation and conclusions of the report. The larger lesson here is the need to avoid overreacting to bioethical innovations, particularly those related to reproductive medicine. At a moment when the president and the public were responding to these developments in emotionally charged ways, it was perhaps the duty of a national bioethics commission to restore some calm to the debate. NBAC tried to do this by producing a report as quickly as possible, but the very effort to do so contributed to the frenzy.

A second criticism concerns the high profile NBAC gave religious views in the testimony and written reports it invited. NBAC's initial meeting on 13–14 March 1997 focused heavily on invited presentations and papers from theologians and ethicists who were explicitly chosen to speak from the perspectives of their religious traditions.[254] Scholars from the Protestant, Catholic, Jewish, and Muslim faiths reported on the range of views within their traditions. NBAC also commissioned a scholarly paper to review religious perspectives on the issue.[255]

Certainly, a case can be made, as NBAC tried to do, for considering reli-gious perspectives within the public policy context.[256] Many Americans are influenced by their religious backgrounds. Because of this, simply as a mea-sure of public opinion and of the likely response to any report, religious views are relevant to the work of a federal commission.[257] In addition, nothing within our tradition of separation of church and state requires religious com-munities to silence themselves on matters they believe to be of public con-cern. By giving religious views a formal place in their process, some NBAC members were also seeking to remedy what they regarded as a defect in the work of the Human Embryo Research Panel. NBAC commissioner Alta Charo, who, when serving on the embryo panel, had championed many posi-tions unacceptable to some large religious organizations, now stated that in its approach to cloning NBAC should correct the earlier panel's failure to explic-itly heed religious views.[258]

Despite these considerations, I believe that NBAC crossed a subtle line and set an unfortunate precedent for public policy debate by giving ethicists representing varying religious traditions a privileged role in the commission's deliberations. It is one thing for religious groups to try to influence public debate through the education of their adherents, who then, as citizens, help to form public policy. It is a very different thing to say that the views of spokespeople from organized religious groups will be given a formal position in the hearings of policy panels. This is an invitation for *every* group to assert its presence on the stage of federal policy formation. It opens the door to the very thing our tradition of church-state separation was meant to avoid: con-flicts over which religious views will be heard and who will represent them. It appears that ethicists from evangelical Christian groups were not among those invited to speak before NBAC. These groups will not long tolerate this kind of exclusion. Once it is understood that religious views have a formal place in this context, a host of traditions will step forward to assert their right to participate. Bioethics policy will then become a site for religious conflict and theological disputation. One can imagine future hearings on bioethics policy and legislation becoming a favored arena for larger cultural wars. The geneticist Richard Lewontin points to this problem when, in a published cri-tique of NBAC's report, he states, "By giving a separate and identifiable voice to explicitly religious views the commission has legitimated religious convic-tion as a front on which the issues of sex, reproduction, the definition of the family, and the status of fertilized eggs and fetuses are to be fought."[259]

This problem is compounded by the fact that religious traditions' conserva-tism and resistance to change has become almost uniquely focused on the area of reproduction and sexuality.[260] In the fields of physics and astronomy, for example, most religious communities have abandoned their efforts to de-fend every feature of an outmoded biblical cosmology. But human sexuality and reproduction remain vulnerable to religious efforts to exert control. Furthermore, almost all religious traditions, not just conservative ones, lay claim to this realm. The reasons for this are not hard to understand. The God of the Bible is particularly active in the area of reproduction. God not only brings humanity into existence as sexual beings ("male and female He created them") but does so explicitly for reproductive purposes ("be fruitful and multiply"). God is also depicted throughout biblical texts as intimately involved in the miracles of conception and birth. This makes it tempting for Jewish, Christian, and Muslim thinkers to exert a proprietary interest in the norms governing reproduction.

Because deep values are involved, religious claims often continue to be made long after they have lost any footing in scientific or social fact. Witness how slowly religious communities have responded to the revolutions represented by the development of birth control and the emergence of rapid population growth (some have still not done so). The resistance shown by many organized religious communities to new information regarding the biological bases of homosexuality is another example.[261] A policy review process that foregrounds religious positions lends prestige to religious communities' often unjustified claims to special expertise in this area. It also tends to skew consideration of these issues in an overly negative direction. In fairness, it must be said that NBAC tried to invite a variety of religious views. The final NBAC report pointed out that the commitee's encounter with religious positions revealed significant diversity, with no single "religious view" emerging.[262] Nevertheless, the religious ethicists that appeared before NBAC representing the largest religious faith communities voiced negative views about cloning.[263]

My third criticism concerns NBAC's most important recommendation: that federal legislation be introduced to prohibit any attempt at human cloning, whether in the public or private sector. It is true that this recommendation was carefully constrained. The commission would permit privately funded human cloning research provided it was not intended to lead to the birth of a cloned child. It also recommended a "sunset provision" in any prohibitory legislation to force reconsideration of the issue in the future. But even when limited in these ways, NBAC's recommendation introduced a dangerous new precedent to federal efforts to control life sciences research.[264] In the United States surprisingly little use has been made of federal legislative power to prohibit research or clinical activities generally. Instead, as I indicated in the previous chapter, regulation results from a complex web of restraints. This includes federal human subjects regulations, standards of care established by professional associations, and civil law tort protections against medical malpractice. In the 1970s, in order to secure time to address pressing safety concerns, scientists even arranged a voluntary moratorium to slow recombinant DNA research until safety issues had been resolved. This loose-textured web of restraints has worked well to forestall the most serious effects of risky biological research. This approach also has the advantage of preventing the government from entirely shutting down a promising line of research or halting the development of greatly desired clinical services. Dedicated scientists who believe their research to be safe and important can seek private support. Patients can vote with their dollars by seeking services from private clinics.

Because NBAC feared that a similarly permissive pattern would prevail in the case of cloning, the commission called for a uniform federal ban on any attempt to clone a human being. A federal ban shifts the emphasis from regulation of government funded research to a blanket prohibition of a research area. Instead of inviting the best scientists to assume responsibility for the direction of the field, it drives away responsible researchers and opens the field to less responsible scientists. Even when a ban is carefully crafted, it induces fear and has a chilling effect. Universities and other research institutions, for whom millions of dollars in other funded research might be put at risk, avoid anything likely to invite legal prosecution.[265] Finally, it was probably naïve for NBAC to think that Congress might in the future allow an existing ban on cloning to expire. Once a federal law against any innovation in reproductive medicine is enacted, inertia takes over and the burden falls on those who would alter the status quo. From that moment on, a small number of dedicated opponents can work to keep a prohibition in place. By urging this unprecedented ban on a research area, NBAC opened the door to permanent research obstruction not only in the field of cloning, but in other fields as well.

My fourth criticism concerns NBAC's decision not to make any recommendations about human embryo research as it relates to cloning.[266] Noting that the issue had "recently received careful attention by a National Institutes of Health panel," the NBAC report chose not to "revisit" it in the context of its treatment of cloning.[267] NBAC chose to bypass this issue for a good reason. Following the announcement of the birth of Dolly, voices were being raised in Congress calling for a prohibition of all human embryo research, private as well as public, in order to close the door on human cloning. These legislators opposed not only human cloning, but also all manipulations of the human embryo not to its benefit. They saw the cloning issue as a chance to implement their wider agenda. If NBAC took up the issue of embryo research, it would only encourage the opponents of embryo research to reopen this debate.

Despite this risk, NBAC had to address the issue of embryo research if it was to give credibility to its concerns about harms to children. Recall that the principal reason behind NBAC's call for a ban on human cloning was the unknown risks of the procedure for the child. How could these risks be assessed and reduced? Animal research was imperative, as the NBAC report acknowledged.[268] All new reproductive technologies are first developed using animal models. Researchers must show that an innovative reproductive technology can be used in other mammalian species and result in normal fertilization, fetal development, birth, and healthy survival. But serious limits exist using animal models. Despite many similarities, embryos of different species develop differently. Eventually, a substantial amount of preliminary research would have to be conducted using cloned human embryos not intended for transfer. These embryos would have to be monitored closely following the nuclear transfer procedure to determine whether they were morphologically and chromosomally normal and whether proper gene expression was occurring. Although this research would focus only on the earliest days of development, information gathered in this way would nevertheless be crucial to assessing and minimizing the risks associated with human transfer procedures. This research might also provide the scientific basis for a permanent ban in this area. If it could be shown that cloned embryos not intended for transfer were unavoidably damaged by this procedure, the Richard Seeds of the world and their clients would think twice before trying to apply this technology.

If NBAC's members really believed that the most pressing questions about cloning concerned the resulting child's safety, they had an obligation to stress the need for continued federally funded research in this area. Without federal support, the burden of providing the information needed for a critical review of the federal ban on cloning a child would fall on private research facilities that had few resources for such studies and that were largely exempt from human subjects regulations and other forms of oversight. This means that there was a serious contradiction at the very heart of the NBAC report. Although the commissioners based their call for a ban on the urgent need to protect born children from harm, they failed to recommend the legal and policy changes most needed to assess that risk and ensure that harm did not occur.

Part of the reason for this strategy was the commission's effort to avoid a confrontation with Congress over the issue of embryo research. At a deeper level, however, this pattern of stressing physical risks yet neglecting the recommendations needed to address them suggests to me that NBAC was not entirely serious about its focus on the risk issue. Instead, this was a convenient way of putting aside many of the larger issues raised by cloning, while still finding grounds to ratify the president's call for a moratorium on cloning research. If so, this tells us that politics, rather than careful attention to good bioethics policy, was the unifying theme in the recommendations of the NBAC report.

Ironically, these political concerns seem not to have borne any fruit. NBAC's recommendations (like those of the Human Embryo Research Panel before it) went virtually unheeded, lost in the political wrangling that continues to cloud the cloning issue. Congress did not put any of NBAC's recommendations into effect, and various bills of increasing degrees of severity and scope all died in committee.[269] But in addition to being guilty of political irrelevance, NBAC missed one of the most propitious opportunities for returning embryo research to the public agenda. Eighteen months later, NBAC's inadequate treatment of embryo research would come back to haunt it when the president asked the commission to examine the issue of stem cell research. Eventually, with politics again in mind, it would lurch to the opposite extreme, becoming a champion of federal involvement in this area to a degree unwarranted by the needs of scientific research.

The risk of harming children remains one of the most pressing reasons for involving the federal government in human embryo research. Without federal support, all new reproductive technologies—not just cloning—regularly expose children to unnecessary dangers. NBAC's poor handling of this issue went beyond its politically expedient neglect of human embryo research. My fifth and final criticism of the NBAC cloning report is that the commission also failed to provide an adequate philosophical account of the obligation we have not to harm our children through the techniques used to bring them into being. This obligation is challenged by certain applications of cloning technology. NBAC's response to this challenge was inadequate.

The obligation to avoid harm to children as a result of the new assisted reproductive technologies raises some of the most interesting and perplexing questions in contemporary philosophical ethics. Most of us intuitively feel that we should strive to minimize these harms. This intuition underlay NBAC's recommendation for a cloning moratorium. Years ago, conservative ethicists such as Leon Kass and Paul Ramsey drew on the same intuition in arguing against developing *in vitro* fertilization (IVF).[270] Kass and Ramsey rightly observed that the initial attempts at IVF would be something of a leap into the dark. Even the most extensive and successful preliminary research using other mammals could not ensure that human IVF would not damage a child, possibly in subtle ways that would not be detected until later in life. These risks, they argued, were imposed merely to satisfy the parents' desire for a biologically related child. But in research ethics, it is generally regarded as wrong to expose children to more than minimal risks for others' benefit. This led Kass and Ramsey to the conclusion that all such reproductive research amounted to "unethical experiments on the unborn."

Unfortunately, as obvious as is the duty to avoid harming a child, conceptualizing this poses serious problems when dealing with the new reproductive technologies. One of the very odd things about these technologies is that without them, *the child who is put at risk would not exist.* Consider, for example, the first IVF baby, Louise Brown. Her mother's fallopian tubes were blocked. In the 1970s, when Steptoe and Edwards were trying to develop

IVF, this meant that Mrs. Brown could not have a biologically related child. The first transfer procedure leading to Louise's birth involved unknown risks. Although Steptoe and Edwards did a great deal of animal research and undertook preliminary studies with embryos not intended for transfer, no one could say for sure that some feature of human IVF would not injure the resulting child. Yet, without the first risky transfer procedure, Louise would never have been born. In view of this, even if something had gone wrong, could she really be said to have been harmed by this research?

Normally, in both law and ethics, we think of harming another person as doing something that makes them *worse off* than they were before. If you drive recklessly, strike a pedestrian, and break his leg, you harm him. The accident victim now faces months of painful recuperation and possibly the loss of some function. He has clearly been made worse off than he was before. However, in the odd case of reproductive medicine, the individual who is damaged by a technology is sometimes not obviously made worse off than he or she was before. Imagine that because of the researchers' unavoidably imperfect knowledge, Louise Brown had been born without a leg. This is an even worse injury than the accident victim's is. But the only way Steptoe and Edwards could have avoided it was by stopping their research short of trying to achieve a birth. In that case, Louise would never have been born. Is someone *worse off* being born without a leg than never having been born? Some think the answer is "no," or at least not a clear "yes." If they are right, then it is not certain that Louise would have been harmed. So long as Louise had a "life worth living," so long as she did not prefer dying to staying alive, it seems that no matter how much damage we had inflicted on her by bringing her into existence, she would not have been made "worse off" and therefore not have been harmed.

This conundrum of reproductive ethics has been widely discussed since the philosopher Derek Parfit introduced it into the philosophical literature in the early 1980s in his book *Reason and Persons*.[271] Parfit developed what he called the "nonidentity" problem. He observed that ordinary "person-affecting" notions of harm do not seem to work well in those reproductive cases in which a measure of injury is inseparable from a particular, identifiable child's coming into being. In order to prevent injury, we could choose not to have the child or delay its conception and have some other (nonidentical) child in its place. But if we do this, we cannot easily justify our choice as aimed at trying to benefit *this particular child*, because the consequence of our decision is that *this child* never exists. If we knowingly choose to proceed and conceive a child likely to be born with a birth defect, it is also not clear that, on balance, the child has been harmed by our decision, because *this particular child* would not have been born without this injury. Because most people willingly accept severe losses of function and considerable suffering rather than choosing to die, it becomes difficult to say just how much injury parents can inflict on a child before we can conclude that the child would have been better off never having been born. This suggests that, on balance, no "harm" is done by a reproductive technology needed to bring a child into being, even if that technology leads to the birth of a child with serious physical or mental disabilities.

Because Parfit believed something is intuitively wrong with this conclusion, he tried to develop other ways of understanding parents' responsibilities to their children. He did so by attempting to develop an "impersonal" approach that moves away from a focus on harms or benefits to identifiable people and instead emphasizes our general obligation of beneficence.[272] According to this approach, I do wrong if I bring a child into the world with a lower degree of well-being than some other child I might have had because, in doing so, I fail to increase the net sum of human well-being. Unfortunately, this approach has problems of its own. For example, if I am morally obligated to increase the total *amount* of well-being in the world, it seems that I should increase the *number* of people living, so long as the net sum of well-being is thereby increased. This entails an obligation to expand human populations and have more children. This obligation might continue in force even though each individual's well-being significantly declined as a result.[273] To avoid this conclusion, I might place stress on increasing the *average* well-being of each person, but, then, new problems arise related to childbearing and population policy. Even if a child's life is very satisfactory, I am morally obligated to avoid having it if its prospects are less than the human average, since the child's birth reduces human well-being on average.[274] In other words, if the "person-affecting" accounts of our obligations to our future children run aground on the problem of understanding how an identifiable individual can be harmed by being born, these "impersonal" accounts founder on their indifference to the impact of our choices on real people.

These peculiar problems are not confined to philosophers' discussions. The "no harm" problem has appeared in the legal sphere over the last two decades in relation to the issue of "wrongful life." During the 1970s and 1980s, as medical practitioners became increasingly involved in reproductive procedures and prenatal testing was more widely used, a number of lawsuits were introduced on behalf of children born with serious birth defects caused by the malpractice of medical professionals. One case involved parents who had given birth to a child with Tay-Sachs disease, a fatal genetic disorder marked by progressive neurological degeneration and early death. A testing laboratory mistakenly informed the parents that they were not carriers of the disease. Lawyers sued the laboratory on behalf of the child, arguing that if the parents had been properly informed, they would not have conceived the child.[275] Ordinarily in cases like this, parents first try *wrongful birth* suits, in which they demand compensation for the additional costs and suffering they experience in having to raise a handicapped child. But sometimes, because statutes of limitation expire more quickly in the case of adults than children, these suits are not possible. The parents and attorneys may then sue on behalf of the child itself, arguing that the child would have been better off if it had never been born.

With some qualifications, U.S. and English courts have not accepted the concept of wrongful life.[276] In addition to concerns about the troubling prospect of allowing children to sue their parents for having conceived them, judges have not been convinced that life with a defect, even a terrible childhood disease like Tay-Sachs or Lesch-Nyhan syndrome, is worse than never having lived at all. Tort law aims at returning an injured party to the "rightful" position he or she held before the injury. But the "rightful position" in these types of cases seems to be nonexistence, and it is hard to know how to compare this with an impaired life. In one ruling, a judge articulated this problem by saying, "Ultimately, the plaintiff's complaint is that he would be better off not to have been born. Man, who knows nothing of death or nothingness, cannot possibly know whether this is true."[277] Another judge put the matter this way:

> Whether it is better never to have been born at all than to have been born with even gross deficiencies is a mystery more properly to be left to the philosophers and the theologians. Surely the law can assert no competence to resolve the issue, particularly in view of the very nearly uniform high value which the law and mankind has [sic] placed on human life, rather than its absence.[278]

Despite these rulings, courts have been troubled by the conclusion that a child who is seriously injured as a result of a medical professional's negligence is not harmed in those cases in which, but for the negligence, the child would not have been born. In some instances, courts have sought other tenuously related legal grounds for awarding damages.[279] In one Israeli case, justices openly supported the wrongful life concept.[280]

The practical implications of this problem have also become evident in the cloning debate. In his writings, John Robertson, one of the nation's leading specialists on reproductive law, has applied the work of Parfit and others to the use of new reproductive technologies in general and to cloning in particular.[281] Robertson correctly observes that in some cases, such as when a parent lacks eggs or sperm, cloning may be the only way for a couple to have a genetically related child. In such circumstances, says Robertson, even if the cloning procedure results in serious physical problems for the child (perhaps a shortened life span or disease caused by mutations in the older somatic cell being used), no alternative way exists for *this child* to be.[282] Testifying before NBAC, Robertson drew the practical conclusion of this analysis. "[The] child who would result would not have existed but for the procedure at issue, and [if] the intent there is actually to benefit that child by bringing it into being . . . [this] should be classified as experimentation for [the child's] benefit. . . ."[283]

A sign of how central these seemingly arcane philosophical debates are to the analysis of this and related reproductive issues was that NBAC, in its report on cloning, tried to respond to Robertson's arguments. Rejecting the claim that somatic cell cloning experiments may "benefit" a child who would not otherwise have been born, the NBAC report states:

> This metaphysical argument, in which one is forced to compare existence with non-existence, is problematic. Not only does it require us to compare something unknowable—non-existence—with something else, it also can lead to absurd conclusions if taken to its logical extreme. For example, it would support the argument that there is no degree of pain and suffering that cannot be inflicted on a child, provided that the alternative is never to have been conceived.[284]

This is an odd rejoinder to Robertson's contentions. One may agree with the sentiments behind NBAC's rejection of the nonidentity position, but the argument voiced here, as Robertson noted,[285] is clearly deficient. Rejecting the possibility of comparing existence to nonexistence, NBAC nevertheless opts for nonexistence over impaired existence. Pointing to the extreme conclusions to which the "nonidentity" argument can lead—literally almost no limit on the suffering parents can inflict on a child in order to have it—the commission does not tell us *why* we should reject this conclusion. In fact, NBAC's rejoinder is not an argument at all, but merely an assertion that something is wrong with the "nonidentity/no harm" position.

One cannot fault a public policy document for failing to engage in extensive philosophical discussion. As the bioethicist and public philosopher Dan Brock has observed, it is rarely, if ever, appropriate for a public ethics commission to present a comprehensive moral position in favor of its arguments. Nevertheless, says Brock, such a commission should present "the principle reasons and arguments" that support its policy recommendations.[286] I would add that, even if a commission cannot publicly resolve a difficult moral question central to its work, it should try to provide an indication that some resolution can be achieved. This can take the form of a brief outline of an argument or footnoted references to more complete discussions.[287] The Human Embryo Research Panel tried to do both when it addressed the moral status of the early embryo. NBAC made no similar effort to reply to Robertson's explicit challenge.

To see that something is wrong with the position taken by Robertson, however, consider the following hypothetical case. A couple is planning to start a family. Just as they are about to do so, the woman comes down with the flu.

She calls her obstetrician and asks whether it is advisable to try to become pregnant soon after she recovers. The obstetrician assures her that there is no reason for concern. He has seen nothing in the literature linking flu to birth defects. But assume that he is wrong. Recent articles in his own professional medical journal warn of an association between this strain of flu and an increased incidence of neural tube defects. Misinformed, the woman proceeds to become pregnant. Nine months later, she gives birth to a girl with spina bifida, a serious injury of the spinal cord. The child is physically handicapped for life.

Because of the obstetrician's neglect of his responsibility to stay up-to-date in his field, especially when an explicit question was asked, the family must now face the burden of raising a disabled child. The child seems clearly to have been injured by this sequence of events. She must go through life with major disabilities. Nevertheless, according to the Parfit/Robertson "nonidentity" position, we cannot say that *this* child has been harmed. If the mother had been properly informed, she might have waited several weeks before trying to become pregnant. In that case, it is almost certain that a different egg and a different sperm would have been involved in the conception. Some other child—not *this* child—would have been born. The existing child thus owes its life to the obstetrician's mistake. Unless a point is reached where the child's suffering and pain are so great that that she would honestly prefer never to have lived, the "nonidentity" account tells us that the child has not been made "worse off" by, and perhaps should even be grateful for, the medical blunder that led to her birth.

If we are uncomfortable with this conclusion, we need to seek a better way of understanding our intuitions and reasoning. To do this, we should return to a central question in the debate. What is it that constitutes harm to a human being? Along with most civil tort law, the Parfit/Robertson approach tells us that we have been harmed when we are made "worse off" by another's actions (or negligence) than we were before. This is usually a reasonable assumption, but it poses problems, as we have seen, when the "before" situation is the imponderable state of never having been.

One way to correct this line of reasoning and arrive at more intuitively acceptable conclusions is to recognize that standard "before-after" comparisons were not designed for these preconception or prebirth situations. This would at least free us from the need to conclude that the child with spina bifida has not been harmed. The fact is that, lacking much knowledge or control of birth outcomes, we have never really had to think about these situations before. The new reproductive technologies have changed all this. We can now predict and prevent congenital defects and reduce their incidence in ways never before possible. With this new power comes new moral responsibility. Not to try to reduce harms to our children seems morally irresponsible. Nevertheless, our standard account of harm as involving a "before-after" worsening of someone's situation either does not apply well to these novel choices or leads to odd conclusions.

We can also go further and try to reconsider and refine our concept of harm in the light of these new possibilities. First, we should be careful to avoid linguistic mirages like those produced when we equate the state of "never having been" with "dying," as is sometimes done in this context. We are averse to dying because, by living, we become a recognizable center of value to others and ourselves. But one who has never lived is not a center of value to anyone. We do not usually regard the children we fail to conceive as being harmed by us, and, apart from certain religious traditions with special theological norms, few people today believe that parents have an obligation to have as many children as they possibly can. This indicates that "never having been conceived" is not a state to which any negative value can be ascribed. In the words of bioethicist Cynthia Cohen, nonexistence before life, unlike death, is "neither good nor bad."[288] It is also inappropriate to use this state of nonexistence in any comparative ways at all. No value, whether positive or negative, should be attached to this state, and it should not be compared with any resulting circumstance of one's life.

How, then, can one harm a child by bringing her into existence with avoidable disabilities or states of suffering? What sense can be made of our hunch that, in some way, at least, this child has been made "worse off" by malpractice or negligence? This question at the heart of the non-identity and wrongful life problems was ignored by NBAC but it demands a reasoned answer. In trying to provide one we might begin by recognizing that even existing judgments about harm do not always exactly fit a simple "before-after" model. We find an interesting illustration of this point in an area of tort law known as "misrepresentation law." A party is sometimes judged as having been harmed not only when they are made worse off than they were before, but also when their reasonable expectations have not been met. For example, in the case of fraudulent investment schemes, courts have sometimes awarded investors not just the money they lost in the scheme, but the monetary returns they *would have received* if the promised gains had materialized. In some instances, the fraudulent scheme has in fact made investors "better off" in absolute terms than they were before, but they are regarded as having suffered damage because their real gains fell far short of what they were promised. This approach to the awarding of damages recognizes that losses created by misrepresentation can include both frustrated expectations and the costs of opportunities forgone. The comparison here is not to the investors' previous states, but to the mental expectations that were created and that continue to exist in the investors' minds.

The idea that people can be harmed not only when they are made worse off in a literal sense but also when others disappoint their reasonable expectations may help explain some of our feelings about these odd, birth-related, wrongful life cases. The paradigm of defrauded expectations applies most directly to the parents in the spina bifida case. They acted on the expectation of the birth of a healthy child. Had they been properly informed, they would have postponed the start of their family by a matter of weeks and probably would have had a healthy child. Because of the doctor's incompetence, their reasonable expectation was dashed. They face a lifetime of material and emotional burdens for which they deserve compensation.

In a slightly different way, the same can be said of the child. When she becomes capable of understanding what happened to her, she might reasonably say, "But for that obstetrician's incompetence, I would not have been paralyzed and would have had a more normal life." In saying this, she would be comparing her current state with the state of the child her parents intended to have and would have had if her mother had received proper advice and postponed conception. In strict terms, of course, *this* living child would never have been *that* other child. Any child born later to her parents would have had a slightly different genetic constitution.[289] Yet the child is not being frivolous in making this comparison. So long as the child is alive, both her parents and the child will reasonably compare her life to that of the child she might have been but for the doctor's negligence. That "intended/expected child," therefore, and not the "never-conceived child," is the relevant comparison for one's thinking about what went wrong. It is this reasonably intended/expected child that defines both the parents' and the child's "rightful position" against which comparisons should be made when we conclude they have been made "worse off."

Let me generalize this point. Parents ordinarily wish to have a healthy child. When a medical professional's incompetence leads to their child being born with a significant disability, they have been disappointed in that expectation. They compare the child they have with the child they reasonably expected to have, and they demand compensation for the difference, just as they would expect compensation if a pediatrician wrongly prescribed a drug to a healthy living child and injured it. In terms of their reasonable expectations, it makes no difference whether the injury is done to an already living child, a fetus, or a child not yet conceived. The comparison is never with nonexistence but with the intended/reasonably expected healthy child.

The same is true, I believe, regarding the child's own perception of her situation. Throughout her life, the child reasonably compares her existence, not with the state of never having been, but with the health conditions of other children around her. These other children roughly define the health status available to children under normal circumstances of birth. In most cases, a child's health condition is beyond anyone's control. Many congenital problems occur for unknown reasons, and a seriously disabled child, although frequently making such comparisons, may look on her condition as a misfortune with which she must live. But when the quality of a child's health at birth is within other people's control, the child reasonably feels harmed if these adults did not take steps to see that she was born with roughly the same prospects as others. To the now-living child, it makes no difference that she would not have been born but for some adult's careless or irresponsible conduct. Had she never been born, she would not be making any comparisons at all. But now that she is alive, she is doing just that, and her comparisons are to that other, healthy living child she might have been. If the adult responsible for this circumstance is a medical professional who has neglected some duty of care, the child may rightly feel injured by this neglect. The same may be true when a parent, through reasonably avoidable behavior, injures a child. This can occur before conception, when, for example, an HIV-infected woman knowingly becomes pregnant or when a woman carelessly disregards information about the link between folic acid deficiency and birth defects. It can also occur after conception through substance abuse leading to fetal alcohol syndrome or when a man beats his pregnant partner and injures their child. In all of these cases, an informed child (become adult) can reasonably say, "I have been harmed. But for my parent's negligence or misconduct, I would have been born healthy."

Obviously, complexities abound in this line of reasoning. Sometimes people cannot possibly have a child without inflicting some injury on it. This is true of those who suffer from some kinds of genetic disorders. Although alternatives exists for such people—adoption or sperm and egg donation—we do not usually think they can be blamed for trying to have a biologically related child. One way of understanding this is to follow the logic of the nonidentity position and say that people never inflict harm on a child when this is the only way of bringing it into being. However, this approach leads back to all the problems I have signaled. Alternatively, we can say that in an era of reproductive control, parents and medical professionals ordinarily have a duty, within the range of their ability, to see to it that a child is born unimpaired and with roughly the same health prospects as other children around it. Failure to exercise this duty harms the child. But this duty to avoid harm to a child is only one important star in the moral firmament. Another is the parents' right not to have others impede them in their effort to have a biologically related child. If the only way they can have a child is by risking its birth with a defect, then it is not always clearly wrong for them to try to do so. Moral choice usually involves a balancing of competing rights and claims. U.S. courts have long recognized this in decisions permitting parents to determine their child's religion, place of residence, and educational opportunities.

Out of respect for the religious beliefs of Amish parents, for example, the Supreme Court has permitted them to significantly limit their children's educational opportunities.[290] In the area of reproductive choices, the court has ruled that employers cannot bar fertile female employees from jobs involving lead exposure. The rights of women to employment, the court ruled, take precedence in this instance over the objective of protecting the children born to these women from the risk of congenital injuries.[291] Sometimes, when the relative weighting of these competing values differs, the balance tilts the other way. U.S. law prohibits Jehovah's Witnesses from denying lifesaving blood transfusions to their children. The assumption is that risk of death is a graver evil than the parents' loss of liberty to determine their child's religion.

Thus, we can understand reproductive choices today as involving a tension between the parents' right not to be impeded in their efforts to have a biologically related child and the child's right not to be born with preventable congenital anomalies that render its health prospects significantly less than those of the other children with whom it is born and among whom it is likely to live.[292] It is this comparative health status, not the state of never having been conceived or born, that is the child's "rightful position" against which its actual condition should be measured in cases of medical malpractice and parental negligence. Using the familiar language of moral rights, we can say that a child has a *prima facie* right not to be born with readily preventable birth defects. This means the right exerts a force on our thinking and must always be weighed against the competing *prima facie* rights of others.

How does this argument apply to the cloning debate? The first efforts at cloning will unavoidably involve some risk to the child's health, both in physiological and psychological terms. Other things being equal, it is wrong to bring children into the world in such circumstances. However, people also have a right not to be impeded in their efforts to have biologically related children. This becomes particularly acute in the case of people who cannot have such a child without cloning. Couples in which one or both partners lack gametes are the most obvious case. Lesbian couples are also likely to be among those who wish to avail themselves of this technology. They have the option of sperm donation, but they may justifiably feel that the use of donor sperm introduces a third party into the relationship, with ensuing emotional and social complications. In these cases, cloning may be a reasonable way for people to fulfill their desire for a biologically related child.

However, if what I have been saying is right, the child's welfare also enters into our moral calculations. On the basis of its reasonable expectations, it has a right to a roughly normal health situation. This means that the actual cloning of a human being should not be undertaken until reasonable confidence exists that the resulting child will not be exposed to unusual physical or psychological risks. Physical risks can be understood and minimized through appropriate prior animal research and human embryo research. Psychological risks can be reduced through careful selection and counseling of prospective parents as well as systematic follow-up of the earliest cloned children.

Hence, NBAC's basic conclusion was right. We should postpone the actual cloning of a human until the physiological risks are well understood and reduced. A delay in cloning will also give us time to reflect on and prepare for possible psychological and social risks associated with this technology. But to say this is not to approve of NBAC's treatment of the issue. On a philosophical level NBAC failed to offer a compelling argument for its focus on physiological risks. As a work of public philosophy, the NBAC report on cloning is deficient. Having stressed the need to ensure the safety of children produced by this procedure, NBAC provided neither the rationale for this recommendation nor the strong support for the embryo research that is needed to implement it.

This philosophical detour into the subject of harm to still unconceived children provides another illustration of a point I have tried to make throughout this book. Rapid advances in biomedical science and technology, particularly at the beginnings of life, are forcing us to reconsider our accustomed ways of thinking about ethical issues in this area. We considered this point in chapters 1 and 2 when I emphasized how our greatly increased knowledge of fertilization and embryogenesis has forced us to perceive the role of choice in all our boundary determinations about moral protectedness. No longer passive discoverers of morally significant markers, we now see clearly that we must choose the points at which moral protection begins and ends.

Similarly, the issue of harm to the unconceived or unborn forces a reconsideration of older ways of thinking. In law and ethics, harm has usually meant making someone worse off than they were before. But the unparalleled control available now at the beginning of life challenges this older notion. In reproductive cases in which the child would never have been born, no measurable "before" is relevant. Nevertheless, our solid intuition that birth with an avoidable defect is undesirable, and our sense that the harmful effects of malpractice and negligence should never be excused, challenge us to rethink this older idea of harm. Searching for resources within legal and moral thinking to help broaden our approach to the issue, we note that harm has sometimes been thought of as extending to the frustration of one's reasonable expectations. This allows us to see that the older "before-after" notion is merely a special case within a broader category of harms interpreted as injuries to real persons that we wish to avoid. Applying this category to children born with preventable birth defects, we develop a more relevant measure by comparing their situation to the child "they reasonably might have been."

I do not mean to suggest that science and technology have changed our most basic ways of thinking about ethics. Fundamentally, I believe, moral choice always involves impartial, rational decision by all members of society regarding the rules of conduct they are willing to accept and obey.[293] What science and technology are showing us, however, is that we must occasionally return to these basic notions and leave behind the crystallized results of previous applications. Confronting older borderlines for life's beginning or end, which have been made less compelling by science and technology, we must use impartial reasoning to redraw our boundaries in more satisfactory ways. Faced in law and ethics with an older notion of harm that no longer deters negligence or protects children, we must seek the underlying conceptions that led us to employ these notions in the first place. In the next chapter, I offer one final illustration of this process: the way cell biology is altering our understanding of the role of "potentiality" in moral arguments at the beginning of life.

7

THE STEM CELL
DEBATE

JUST when it seemed that federal support for human embryo research
would never materialize because of Congress's opposition and NBAC's silence, the issue reappeared explosively in November 1998. John Gearhart of
the Johns Hopkins University and James Thomson of the University of Wisconsin published papers in two leading science journals announcing that their
research teams had created immortalized human stem cell lines.[294] Gearhart
had used tissues from aborted fetuses; Thomson's group had derived their cell
line by dissecting spare human embryos from infertility procedures.

In two respects, the Human Embryo Research Panel's report had proved
prophetic. Thanks to science co-chair Brigid Hogan, we gave substantial attention to human stem cell research and offered several recommendations.
We placed the creation of immortalized stem cell lines from spare embryos in
our category of "acceptable research." After a long series of debates, we remained divided on the question of whether researchers should be permitted
to create research embryos for this purpose, voting narrowly to put the matter
in the category of "warranting additional review." Most of the panel members
would have preferred to declare this research "acceptable," while a smaller
number wanted to rule it out entirely.[295]

The report proved prophetic in a second sense. We said that the refusal of
federal funding would not stop human embryo research but would, instead,

merely drive it into private hands. This is exactly what had happened. In return for exclusive licensing of the technologies that Gearhart and Thomson developed, the Geron Corporation of Menlo Park, Calif., had supported their work.[296] This did not mean there was to be no ethical oversight of the research. Each scientist chose to use his university's institutional review board (IRB) process to examine the implications of the research for human subjects.[297] In addition, Geron set up its own ethics advisory board (EAB) to provide guidance for its involvement in this area. Following the announcement of Gearhart's and Thomson's research, the Geron EAB issued a brief statement that had been finalized the previous month affirming that research on stem cells derived from human embryos could be conducted ethically.[298] Geron-funded research, it said, is conducted within the guidelines established by the 1994 NIH Human Embryo Research Panel Report and the 1997 National Bioethics Advisory Committee report (presumably, the NBAC report on cloning). Members of the advisory board, it continued, were unanimous in taking a developmental view of the moral status of early human life. They agreed that, although "the blastocyst must be treated with the respect appropriate to early human embryonic tissue," its use in research could be justified when that research "aims ultimately to save or heal human life."

Despite these efforts, critics were quick to note the limits of Geron's in-house EAB.[299] Although efforts had been made to reduce the corporation's influence on its members (they were paid only modest fees for their service), this was still not an authoritative, governmental oversight body.[300] In a critical article, my embryo panel colleague Carol Tauer observed that the advisory board's guidelines seemed to have been formulated *after* Gearhart and Thomson conducted the bulk of their research.[301] Just as the embryo panel had predicted, in other words, the opportunity to conduct stem cell research and the government's forced abandonment of funding in this area had given rise to an ambitious private sector research effort the ethical review of which raised questions.

A further problem would manifest itself only with time. This was the prospect of Geron gaining a commercial monopoly of the entire area of stem cell research. Although Geron's president, Thomas Okarma, publicly affirmed that the corporation would make immortalized stem cell lines and related technologies available "at cost" to other researchers, this was only part of the picture. "Pass through" agreements, which Geron would surely require, would give the company a share in commercial benefits of downstream applications resulting from its basic stem cell technology. In 1999 Geron purchased Roslin Bio-Med, the commercial arm of the Roslin Institute. This was part of a long-term strategy to acquire patents on the cloning technologies needed for the development of autologous (immunologically compatible) human stem cell lines for therapeutic purposes.[302] In short, Geron was positioning itself to be a major toll-keeper on the biotech highway it was helping to build.

The research had enormous potential value in both medical and commercial terms. Stem cells are the progenitors of all specialized cells in the body. Blood stem cells (hematopoietic cells) reside in bone marrow and continuously produce a variety of blood and immune system cells. Mesenchymal stem cells are the source of new bone, cartilage, and connective tissue cells. Neuronal stem cells produce a variety of nervous system tissue, mostly during early embryonic development but, as we are beginning to learn, later in life as well. During early development, the precursors to all these more specialized stem cells, sometimes called "pluripotential stem cells" (PSCs), are found in the inner cell mass of the preimplantation embryo and in certain cell populations of the early fetus.

Thomson and Gearhart, using different approaches, had isolated these very early precursor cells and spread them out on a feeder layer of mouse cells to produce an immortalized pluripotent human stem cell culture. Research showed that the resulting cell lines produce the enzyme telomerase, which resets the cells' chromosomal clocks and prevents the timed death suffered by most differentiated cells. This resetting allows the cells to be cultured indefinitely during repeated cell divisions (or passages). In the future, when better understanding has been gained of the growth factors that induce specific forms of cell differentiation, immortalized PSC lines like these may be induced to produce specific tissue types. It would then be possible to generate in the laboratory insulin-producing islet cells to cure diabetes or dopamine-producing cells the absence of which causes Parkinson's disease. Also on the distant horizon lies the possibility of new cardiac tissue for heart attack victims, replacement blood and marrow cells for those who have undergone chemotherapy or radiation therapy for cancer, new skin tissue for burn victims, bone for those suffering from severe fractures or osteoporosis, and so on. Closely studied, stem cell lines might give scientists new clues about the growth factors that drive tissue differentiation from the earliest embryonic stage forward. This would permit new understanding of cellular abnormalities, including cancer, and new ways of steering cell differentiation in desired paths. Thomas Okarma articulated Geron's corporate hope and a likely reality when he predicted that in the twenty-first century, cell replacement therapies based on pluripotent stem cell lines will render obsolete many current drug and medical interventions.[303] At the end of 1999, the journal *Science*, in a special cover article and editorial, declared pluripotent stem cell research to be the scientific "breakthrough" of the year.[304]

Major legal, ethical, and political hurdles stand in the way of these advances. In large part, these obstacles result from the fact that, of the three sources of stem cells, human embryos are the most promising. One source is the "adult," or mature, stem cells that reside in the body from infancy onward. These cells are "multipotent," meaning they are able to produce a range of related tissues, such as the differing types of blood system cells. A second source is embryonic germ (EG) cells that are derived from the primordial reproductive tissues of aborted early fetuses. These are the cells that John Gearhart used in his research. They are pluripotent, able to give rise to all tissue types, although recent research suggests that their usefulness in cell replacement therapies might be limited because they have already begun to take on some specific characteristics of their reproductive function.[305] Finally, there are embryonic stem (ES) cells, derived from the inner cell mass of blastocyst-stage embryos. These pluripotent cells are the most ubiquitous of all. Once removed from the blastocyst they lack the outer trophoblast structures needed for continued embryonic development, but they can theoretically be "nudged" into becoming any cell type found in the human body. These are the cells that Thomson used in his research.

Publication of Thomson's and Gearhart's studies made the issue of federal support for human embryo research unavoidable. Gearhart's use of tissue from aborted fetuses could be federally funded because research using cadaveric fetal tissue is currently not prohibited by federal law.[306] However, Thomson's use of spare human embryos provided by the University of Wisconsin's infertility clinic would be a direct violation of the existing ban on federally-funded human embryo research. In order not to imperil the university's massive budget of government-supported research, Thomson set up a separate lab in a building across campus from where he did his NIH-funded research.[307]

Within days of the publication of Thomson's and Gearhart's papers, efforts were underway to review the impact of the existing ban on future federal support for such research. President Clinton once again instructed NBAC to review the matter and report back to him with recommendations.[308] The NIH set up a special small ad hoc subcommittee to consider the matter. That subcommittee, which reported to the Advisory Committee to the Director (ACD), included Human Embryo Research Panel members Brigid Hogan and Carol Tauer. The NIH's legal counsel also set about reviewing pluripotent stem cell research in light of existing laws and regulations. By early 1999, Congress was holding hearings on the issue, members of Congress and senators were signing petitions, and Harold Varmus and Richard Doerflinger were once again preparing testimony and issuing statements. In terms of embryo research, we had come full circle to the events of 1994.

Three issues spurred the debate. One concerned the moral status of PSCs themselves. Are they morally protectable entities, or are they more like other disposable tissues gleaned from the human body? A second issue concerned the derivation of PSCs. Assuming that at least during the earliest phases of research, human embryos produced via *in vitro* fertilization (IVF) would be the best source for producing immortalized stem cell lines, could research go forward that depended on the dissection of living human embryos? These questions had both legal and ethical dimensions. Whatever the rightness or wrongness of pluripotent stem cell use or embryo destruction, the Dickey-Wicker amendment prohibited funding for "research in which a human embryo or embryos are destroyed." In light of this ban, could the NIH enter the field, or must it continue to leave it to private researchers?

Finally, there was the question, still somewhat remote but now looming, that had preoccupied us on the embryo panel: whether to permit the creation of research embryos. For cell replacement therapies to fulfill their promise, cell lines must be produced that can overcome rejection by the recipient's immune system. The hope is that we will develop enough knowledge to do this by manipulating the immune system factors of standardized pluripotent stem cell lines. If this is not possible, each therapeutic intervention will require the preparation of tissues that are immunologically suitable (histocompatible) for the patient. One way to do this might be to combine Thomson's stem cell work with the cloning technology developed by Ian Wilmut and his colleagues at the Roslin Institute. A somatic cell could be taken from the recipient individual, its nucleus inserted into an enucleated egg cell that is stimulated to begin dividing, and the resulting blastocyst-stage embryo then disaggregated to produce a histocompatible pluripotent stem cell line. The prospect of this union of pluripotent stem cell and cloning technology is one reason why early in 1999 Geron acquired the Roslin Institute, along with its cloning patents.

If this scenario of therapeutic (as opposed to reproductive) cloning is realized, the deliberate creation of human embryos will become a routine part of clinical care. Ways around this exist, but they only compound the ethical problems. In early 1999, Advanced Cell Technology, a Worcester, Mass., company headed by Michael West, one of the founders of Geron, announced that it was working on a therapeutic cloning technology that used cow oocytes as the source of enucleated eggs.[309] This approach reduced reliance on scarce human eggs. It also meant that the resulting embryos were not exactly *human*. However, the Human Embryo Research Panel had placed the development of human–nonhuman chimeras (with or without transfer) in our category of unacceptable research.[310] Admittedly, this was not one of our more carefully considered recommendations. It was a result of weariness at the end of extensive deliberations, a sense that this possibility was too distant to merit serious consideration, and an unreflective emotional reaction to the creation of quasi-human "monsters." Now pluripotent stem cell research was challenging that inattention and placing the two controversial issues of research embryos and chimeras back on the public agenda.

During much of the winter of 1999, I was on the sidelines as this national debate got underway. My wife was teaching a Dartmouth foreign study program in Toulouse, France. I had a free term and had accompanied her to finish some writing. One evening in late January, I received a telephone call from Gina Kolata, a leading science writer for *The New York Times*. The NIH legal counsel had just issued the opinion that human pluripotent stem cells were not "embryos." This view was based, in part, on the fact that, by themselves, pluripotent stem cells cannot perform all the functions of life, including generation of the placental structures needed for further development. Yet Kolata noted that, six years earlier, a team of Canadian researchers headed by Andràs Nagy at the University of Toronto had grown entire mice from individual stem cells they had plucked from a mouse embryo.[311] They did this by injecting the stem cells into an existing embryo whose own cells were genetically engineered to self-destruct in a short period of time. The mouse that was eventually born was composed entirely of cells derived from the inserted stem cells. "Didn't this call into question the claim that stem cells cannot become a human being?" Kolata asked me.

I did not offer an opinion about the status of stem cells, but others who were quoted in the story, which appeared on 9 February, did. John Gearhart and Brigid Hogan denied that stem cells are like embryos, pointing to their inherent lack of ability to develop into a full person. Lee Silver, a mouse biologist at Princeton who has taken controversial stands on many reproductive and genetic issues, rejected that view. If what matters is the capacity to develop into a human being, he said, "then human embryonic stem cells are the moral equivalent of embryos. Metaphysically, it's all the same."[312]

My more general reply grew out of my deepest beliefs about how we should think about determining the moral status of entities. I pointed out that in an era of cloning, every cell in the human body has the potential to become a complete human being. If we accept the conclusion that all these cells are "potential people," it will have profound implications for every aspect of human life. Whatever route we take, we will not get there by definitions or simple appeals to biological "facts." "The problem," I observed, "is that people are still trying to use biology to draw moral lines in the sand, and biology just does not suffice anymore. . . . The biology only poses decisions."

Within a few weeks, my distance from these debates would end and I would once again have to put this basic understanding to work. In March, when I had returned from France, I received an invitation from Audrey Chapman and Mark Frankel of the American Association for the Advancement of Science (AAAS) to participate in a working group on the issue of pluripotent stem cell research. The AAAS is one of the most prestigious organizations of scientists in the world. Audrey, whose background was in religious ethics, headed up the association's Program of Dialogue Between Science and Religion; Mark was director of the Scientific Freedom, Responsibility and Law Program. Audrey and Mark believed that AAAS owed its members and the country a scientifically and ethically informed contribution to the growing national debate. Collaborating with the Institute for Civil Society, a group dedicated to fostering public discourse, they hoped to prepare a document that, along with NBAC's pending report, would influence public discussion and congressional action.

The working group met for the first time at AAAS headquarters in Washington on 7–8 April 1999. In addition to Audrey and Mark from AAAS and Gail Pressburg from the Institute for Civil Society, 17 members were present. I was pleased to find myself once again involved in the kind of multidisciplinary panel that I believe is essential to the formation of good public policy in bioethics. The members included scientists from both the university and private sectors. Among them were Robert Goldman, a cell biologist from Northwestern University Medical School; David Gottlieb, a neurobiologist at Washington University in St. Louis; and Daniel Marshak, chief scientific officer of Osiris Therapeutics, a Maryland-based company that was trying to develop and commercialize mesenchymal stem cell lines. Bioethicists were well represented. They included Courtney Campbell, former editor of the *Hastings Center Report* and now teaching at Oregon State University; Dena Davis, an ethicist and lawyer at Cleveland-Marshall School of Law, whom I had known since her student days at Vermont's Marlboro College; Cynthia Cohen, a senior research fellow at Georgetown's Kennedy Institute of Ethics; Abigail Evans of the Princeton Theological Seminary; Kevin Fitzgerald of Loyola University in Chicago; Norman Fost, who directed the medical ethics program at the University of Wisconsin, where James Thomson had done his research; C. Ben Mitchell of the Southern Baptist Theological Seminary in Louisville, Kentucky; and Robert Wachbroit, a philosopher at the University of Maryland at College Park, with whom I had worked and whose abilities I had come to respect during my NIH service. Andrea Bonnicksen, a political scientist from Northern Illinois University, who had written a paper for the Human Embryo Research Panel, offered a policy perspective. The group was rounded out by representatives of several organizations and associations with special interests in our topic. They included David Byers, executive director of the Committee on Science and Human Values of the National Conference of Catholic Bishops; Robert Goldstein, vice-president for research at the Juvenile Diabetes Foundation; Daniel Perry, executive director of the Washington-based Alliance for Aging Research; and Gillian Woollett, vice-president for biologics and biotechnology at the Pharmaceutical Research and Manufacturers of America (PhRMA).

My sense of déjà vu was amplified by our first day's proceedings. As had been true at meetings of the embryo panel, science presentations alternated with policy overviews. NIH concerns and interests also occupied a good part of our time. Lana Skirboll of the NIH Office of Science Policy (the same office that had organized the Human Embryo Research Panel) was invited to outline the legal position with which the NIH was becoming identified. This position was laid out in a memo to Harold Varmus that was prepared by Harriet S. Rabb of the Office of General Counsel of the Department of Health and Human Services (HHS). The memo offered the opinion that the statutory prohibition on funding for human embryo research "would not apply to research utilizing human pluripotential stem cells because such cells are not a human embryo within the statutory definition."[313]

Within this brief statement, two distinct issues were somewhat confusedly addressed. The first concerned the question of whether the NIH could fund research that *used* pluripotent stem cell lines that the researcher had not been involved in deriving. This issue was not explored further in the memo, but it would nevertheless move to the fore in the weeks and months ahead as the NIH struggled to find some elbowroom for supporting pluripotent stem cell research within statutory limitations. The second and more obvious issue concerned the status of stem cells, however they were derived. The memo went on to take the position that pluripotent stem cells should not be thought of as "embryos" within the language of the existing statute. Citing the most recent annual appropriations act to which the prohibition was attached,[314] the memo pointed to the statutory definition of an embryo as "any organism . . . that is derived by fertilization, parthenogenesis, cloning, or any other means from one or more human gametes or human diploid cells."

A key question, the memo observed, is whether a pluripotent stem cell is an "organism." Since the statute does not define this term, the memo sought to address the question with a "science-based answer." Referring to the definition of an organism in the *McGraw-Hill Dictionary of Scientific and Medical Terms* as "[a]n individual constituted to carry out all life functions,"[315] the memo concluded that pluripotent stem cells "are not organisms and do not have the capacity to develop into an organism that could perform all the life functions of a human being—in this sense they are not even precursors of human organisms." The memo also denied that stem cells should be understood as embryos on any other grounds. A human embryo, it held, "has the potential to develop in the normal course of events into a living human being." But pluripotent stem cells "do not have the capacity to develop into a human being, even if transferred to a uterus." On all of these counts, stem cells should be regarded as human cells with, at most, the potential to develop into different cell types.

Most of the memo's attention was given to this treatment of the status of stem cells. But important questions remained to be asked about the first issue: the *use* of stem cells derived from living human embryos that must be destroyed in order to produce the stem cell lines. Would a "downstream" NIH-funded scientist using one of these lines be engaged in research "in which a human embryo or embryos are destroyed"? The Rabb memo gave no explicit answer, although one was suggested by its conclusion that "federally funded research that utilizes human pluripotent stem cells would not be prohibited by the HHS appropriations law prohibiting human embryo research."[316] The key word here is "utilizes." The NIH was envisioning a scenario in which research *using* immortalized pluripotent stem cell lines would be funded by the government but the *derivation* of those lines would be left to private funding. The federally funded component would not be research "in which an embryo or embryos are destroyed," not only because stem cells are not embryos, but because federally funded researchers would merely use established cell lines and would not themselves be involved in destroying embryos. The destruction of embryos would occur earlier, under private auspices.

Shortly after the release of the Rabb memo, the NIH made it explicit that it was considering funding research using, but not deriving, ES cell lines. That distinction became an immediate source of controversy. By early February seventy members of the House and seven senators signed letters to HHS Secretary Donna Shalala protesting the NIH's plans. The House letter declared that the NIH's (Rabb's) interpretation violated "both the letter and spirit" of the law that banned federal funding for destructive embryo research. This law, the letter continued, does not merely prohibit "the act of destroying an embryo." It also bars the use of tax dollars to fund research "which follows or depends upon the destruction of or injury to a human embryo."[317] In the weeks and months ahead, this issue of derivation versus use would become the most divisive ethical and legal issue in the continuing debate.

The issue was no less controversial among the members of our AAAS working group. Several responded to Lana Skirboll's presentation with skepticism. Norm Fost was sharpest in his criticism. He did not object to embryo destruction. Indeed, he was chair of the Bioethics Advisory Committee at the University of Wisconsin that had unanimously declared Thomson's work to be ethically acceptable. What he objected to was what he regarded as a morally dubious separation of the researcher from the acts that made the research possible. It would be more honest and ethically consistent, Fost believed, to argue for the legitimacy of using *and* deriving ES cells.

I was initially sympathetic to Fost's criticisms, but I would soon change my mind. My first, instinctive response was partly a result of the sketchy and oblique way the Rabb memo treated the subject. It also stemmed from the fact that the working group had not yet had time to closely examine the ethical, legal, and political ramifications of the problem. Superficially, we seemed to be faced with an extension of the position that the humorist Tom Lehrer spoofs in his song about the German rocket scientist Werner von Braun: "'When the rockets go up, I don't care where they come down. It's not my department,' says Werner von Braun." To some of us, it seemed that we were now hearing, "'We just use embryos; we don't care where they come from. It's not our department,' says the NIH."

The second day of our first meeting gave us a chance to discuss various sides of these issues among ourselves. At the close of the day, Audrey and Mark formed subgroups that would prepare draft chapters of a report. Once again I found myself on an ethics subgroup with the special assignment of developing a position on the moral status of pluripotent stem cells. Bob Wachbroit, Dena Davis, and I were also charged with looking at the question of whether it is ethically possible to use established pluripotent stem cell lines without becoming ethically complicitous in the destructive acts needed to produce them. Dena would develop guidelines to insure informed consent by those individuals or couples who might provide embryos for ES cell research. Other subgroups were asked to address the scientific, religious and spiritual, and regulatory issues.

Over the next few weeks, portions of chapters began to emerge out of a barrage of e-mail messages. The status of pluripotent stem cells themselves, on which I was focusing, posed relatively few problems. The Rabb memo seemed broadly right. A stem cell is not an "organism" in the sense of being capable on its own of performing all essential life functions. Notably, it lacks the capacity for independent development to adulthood. As a result, even those who regarded the embryo as a human subject because of its potential for development should hesitate before declaring pluripotent stem cells to be morally protectable.

In reality, matters are more complicated, and it is essential to have a solid understanding of *how* these judgments should be made in order to comfortably handle the complexities. Dictionary definitions alone will not suffice. For example, the McGraw-Hill dictionary defines an organism as "[a]n individual constituted to carry out all life functions." But precisely which "life functions" does the dictionary have in mind? Stem cells cannot perform *all* life functions, but with a modicum of support they can divide and propagate themselves indefinitely. In that sense they can perform all the life functions of stem cells. Embryos, too, cannot perform all adult human life functions (they cannot digest food by themselves, move, fight off most threats, and so on), but they can perform the "life functions" appropriate to the embryonic stage of human life, including the function of sustaining metabolism and building support mechanisms for continued growth. Clearly, there is a need within the framework of this definition to determine *which* life functions are significant. Why is an embryo, with its potential for development, to be regarded as a complete organism even at the one cell stage, while a pluripotent stem cell, which lacks this potential but exercises many similar life functions, is not?

Choices and decisions are clearly involved even at this definitional stage, but they were not articulated or made clear by the Rabb memo.

A similar problem arises when we look at the argument from potential. Embryos, the Rabb memo stated, have "the potential to develop in the normal course of events into a living human being." Stem cells lack this capacity. But as Gina Kolata's *New York Times* article had reminded us, scientists have already placed mouse stem cells in an environment where, with some manipulation, they were able to form an adult individual. This cannot be done with differentiated body cells. In addition, evidence exists that stem cells growing in a culture medium sometimes begin to resume embryogenesis, undergoing the beginning of gastrulation and development of the primitive streak.[318] Lacking appropriate supporting structures, however, the cells cannot continue independent development.

Stem cells, too, thus seem to have some potential for development. One might object that this potential would require highly contrived interventions and does not occur "in the normal course of events." But why should the "normal course of events" dictate our thinking on this matter, rather than the mere fact of potential for development, regardless of how it is achieved? In other areas of medicine, a distinction between the "normal course of events" and artificially achieved outcomes is not morally significant. The lives of many classes of people—diabetics, recipients of kidney dialysis, and some AIDS patients—depend on highly contrived interventions. If the "normal course of events" were the baseline for establishing moral entitlements, we might abandon these people as moribund or no longer really alive, but we do not do so. Why, when the distinction between pluripotent stem cells and human embryos is at issue, should "the normal course of events" bear such heavy normative weight in determining what comes within our sphere of protection?

To cut through these confusions and definitional debates, it helps to return to the insight I tried to convey in my discussion in chapter 2 about drawing boundary lines for a moral community. What drives our thinking here are not stipulated definitions or self-evident properties, but urgent practical needs and choices. Status determinations are always moral decisions. They involve careful "balancing judgments" in which we weigh the reasons *for* granting some measure of protection to an entity with certain properties against the reasons for *not* granting it protection. Obviously, the practical implications of protecting any cells with the potential for development are enormous. In an era of cloning, almost all somatic cells have this kind of potentiality. To commit us morally to protecting every living diploid cell in the body would be insane. This practical consideration makes a further "natural-artificial" distinction compelling, especially for those who wish to extend some degree of protection to embryos but not to all somatic cells. By committing ourselves to protecting only cells with "natural" as opposed to "artificial" or "contrived" potentiality, we can greatly limit our moral exposure.

Once we understand this, we can see that it puts things backwards to say that the *reason* embryos are morally protectable but pluripotent stem cells are not is *because of* the distinction between natural and artificially contrived potentiality for development. Rather, the natural-artificial distinction itself comes from a prior moral choice made to avoid an enormously costly commitment to protecting all body cells. It so happens that this distinction has the added benefit of sparing us from having to regard pluripotent stem cells as morally protectable. Because even those who want to protect embryos have to draw lines somewhere, and because no longstanding commitment to stem cells exists, this distinction becomes a useful point for articulating a distinction.

Note that the importance of this distinction between natural and artificially contrived potential once again illustrates the power of scientific and technological change to disrupt our previously established boundary markers, or at least to force a rethinking of them. Until the birth of Dolly, those who wished to defend the importance of a boundary marker at or near conception could articulate their choice (made largely, I believe, on many other grounds) in terms of the zygote's "potential for development into a human being." Cloning has complicated that phrase. Now, one must refine what one means by potentiality. Just as new technologies at the end of life have forced us to determine when we want to say that "death" (as a morally significant event) has occurred, our growing understanding and control of early embryological development has forced us to determine when we want the protections afforded nascent human life to start. In all these cases, science and technology have blurred older boundary lines based on arbitrarily established definitions, imprecise factual understandings, or circumstances in which a limited range of choice was mistaken for the absence of choice.

The second major question before our subgroup was a relatively new one for me, but it proved to be one of the most fascinating—and important—parts of our work. What are the limits of cooperation or complicity with moral evil? When, if ever, may one ethically benefit from or use the results of an activity that were produced by what one regards as morally questionable, or even morally heinous, methods?

I had encountered this question before. One day during my service at the NIH, I received a telephone call from an administrator in the genome institute. She had a peculiar question. Knowing that I was based in a religious studies department and that I was also of Jewish background, she asked, "In the period leading up to the Nazi era, was it customary for non-Jews in Germany or Austria to be circumcised?" I replied that I believed that relatively few non-Jewish Germans or Austrians of that period were circumcised because the Nazis were able to use circumcision as a way to identify Jews seeking to pass as Christians. "Why do you ask?"

She went on to explain that concern had been expressed about a series of illustrated color anatomy texts in the NIH library that had been published in Vienna in the early 1940s. It was believed that the author used as models cadavers supplied by the Gestapo. Several illustrations contained circumcised male genitals, suggesting they may have been based on photos or sketches made of Jewish victims of Nazi persecutions.[319]

The question was whether one should retain and use texts that resulted from moral atrocities. This question had arisen previously in discussions about the use of information gleaned from biomedical research done on concentration camp inmates.[320] But because most of that research was of doubtful scientific value, the discussion was more academic than real. Now an NIH administrator was asking what should be done with a set of exquisitely illustrated anatomy texts still widely used by NIH researchers and physicians.

After thinking the matter over, I offered the opinion that even if the allegations about these texts proved true, it would be wrong to remove them from the library. They are still regarded as a standard in the field and are widely consulted. Censorship for any reason is repugnant. However, I added that it might be a good idea to place in these texts an explanation of their sources as well as references to articles dealing with the controversy. In this way, the existence of the texts would recall and perhaps even honor the victims.

Nazi science was on my mind as I considered the question of whether researchers should use ES cell lines derived from the destruction of human embryos. Normally, I would hesitate to bring these two issues together. Holocaust analogies have too often been misused in debates about embryo research.[321] Furthermore, the analogy is reasonable only if one accepts the troubling premise that human embryos are morally equivalent to the adult and child victims of genocide. Nevertheless, for two reasons it is important when thinking about ES cells to start from this very premise and ask whether research using ES cell lines can be separated from the acts that produce them. First, whether we agree or not, since the passage of the Dickey-Wicker amendment, U.S. law *has* placed the preimplantation embryo on a par with any human subject. As a result, the NIH is legally forbidden to fund any research in which human embryos are destroyed. As the Rabb memo suggests, this leaves open the question of whether a "downstream" NIH-funded researcher who is not involved in the embryo's destruction can use the immortalized pluripotent stem cell lines produced from it. Is this researcher involved in prohibited research "in which" an embryo is destroyed, or is it more correct to say that this researcher innocently benefits from acts performed by others? Does *use* of resulting cells and tissues imply involvement in prohibited acts? Although answering this question requires a careful examination of statutory language, it also involves an unavoidable exercise of judgment about the allowable degree of a government-funded researcher's relationship to legally prohibited acts.

A second reason for assuming in this context that embryos have significant moral status concerns the ethical and political question of how we are to achieve a viable moral consensus on this issue. Many members of society view the early embryo as a fully protectable human being, or at least regard it as important enough that they are not willing to destroy it. Many of these people would presumably oppose using existing ES cell lines unless it could be shown that such use was genuinely, morally separable from the act of embryo destruction. The AAAS working group included one representative of the National Catholic Bishops' Conference and several theologians and ethicists who belonged to religious traditions opposed to abortion. Could these members support a report that recommended research *using* ES cell lines? Was there room for some common ground? Although I profoundly disagreed with the comparisons between embryo research and the Holocaust, my own personal aversion to any use of Nazi research results gave me a point of reference as I tried to understand the struggle occurring in these colleagues' minds. They understood the value of ES cell research. The question remained of how willing they were to accept what they regarded as evil acts in order to produce these benefits.

Bob Wachbroit got our subgroup discussions and writing off to a good start by offering a succinct analysis of the issue of wrongful involvement in moral evil. He noted that philosophical discussions have identified four different ways in which one could become guilty of cooperating with or benefiting from evil. The first is actual, direct involvement in the wrongful deed, as, for example, when a researcher administers a lethal drug dose to an innocent victim in order to collect tissue samples. The second is direct encouragement to evil, as, for example, when researchers encouraged others to kill concentration camp inmates to ensure themselves a supply of research material. The third is indirect encouragement of wrongful killing, as, for example, when researchers perform studies the beneficial consequences of which lead to wider acceptance of wrongful practices and their perpetuation. The fourth, even when encouragement is not an issue, is the appearance of endorsing, conferring legitimacy on, or diluting the condemnation of a wrongful deed.

How did ES cell research measure up on these counts? On an initial review it seemed to do very badly. James Thomson's research violated the first, and arguably the most important, of these criteria. He was directly involved in the dissection and destruction of the spare embryos that were ES cell sources. Thomson's direct involvement in embryo destruction explains why his research had been singled out from the start as a source of ethical and legal concern. Interestingly, far fewer objections were raised to John Gearhart's EG cell research. Gearhart used the tissues of aborted fetuses obtained from a nearby clinic. He played no role in these induced abortions, which were independently requested by the women and performed by clinic personnel. In terms of the first two criteria for wrongful cooperation, he seemed exempt from blame. Did his work violate the third and fourth criteria? Was it reasonable to believe that the possibly beneficial consequences of EG cell research would lead to wider acceptance of abortion? Would it otherwise endorse, confer legitimacy on, or dilute the condemnation of abortion?

During the 1980s, these questions had been extensively reviewed and debated in connection with the issue of fetal tissue transplantation research. The 1988 *Report of the Human Fetal Tissue Transplantation Research Panel* had concluded, with some dissents, that with proper regulation, it is "highly unlikely" that use of tissues from aborted fetuses would encourage women to have an abortion.[322] Women who resorted to abortion did so for reasons unrelated to fetal tissue transplantation research, the report concluded. So long as a woman received no tangible benefit from donating tissue (through payment for fetal tissue or a permission for directed donation of tissues to relatives or loved ones), and an effort was made to separate deliberations and discussion of the abortion decision from the decision to donate tissue, no likelihood existed that fetal tissue research would alter this reality. In essence, the report concluded that researchers using fetal tissue and recipients of that tissue could meet all four criteria for noninvolvement in abortion.

Experience sometimes confirms good moral reasoning. Although the Bush administration did not accept the recommendations of this panel, President Clinton put them into effect by executive order during the first month of his presidency. By 1999, the soundness of the report's recommendations was being upheld on several fronts. Clinical evidence was accumulating for the therapeutic value of fetal tissue transplants for Parkinson's disease, justifying the report's strong support of what had been merely a promising research direction.[323] Public debate had also quieted down. Regulations preventing commercialization or directed donation of fetal tissues apparently had convinced many people of the possibility of morally separating the use of fetal tissues from their derivation. No evidence existed of increased resort to abortion by women seeking to contribute fetal tissue for research. With its attention focused on issues of embryo research, the anti-abortion movement seemed to have moved fetal tissue transplantation research off its most urgent agenda. One sign of this shift was the astonishing introduction late in 1999, right in the middle of congressional debates about stem cell research, of yet another appropriations amendment by Representative Jay Dickey. The congressman was seeking to extend his ban on funding for research in which an embryo is destroyed to include research using ES cell lines. Nevertheless, in a bid to the other side, the amendment explicitly authorized funding for research on adult stem cell lines *and* the type of EG cell research undertaken by John Gear-hart. Within the space of a decade, in other words, fetal tissue research had gone from being a main target of the anti-abortion movement to a research area accepted by one of the movement's principal congressional proponents.

None of these developments improved the prospects for ES cell research. Even though Gearhart's method of deriving pluripotent stem cell lines was now widely viewed as not complicitous with abortion, Thomson's research remained a target of criticism. As I thought about this situation in light of Bob Wachbroit's review of the criteria for evaluating the degree of moral involvement, an idea struck me. I realized that both those in favor of and those opposed to Thomson's research were partly being misled by his exam-ple. His research promoted the assumption that the ES cell researcher must be involved in embryo destruction. But is this really true? In the field of mouse research, I knew, many researchers use widely available immortalized ES cell lines that they acquire from other researchers or from commercial sources and that they play no role at all in deriving. A check with science colleagues on the panel confirmed the conclusion that the bulk of important future research on human ES cell lines would probably involve the use, but not the derivation, of established cell lines. If this is so, most future ES cell researchers would not violate Wachbroit's first criterion: they would not be directly involved in embryo destruction. It remained to be seen how this research would fare in terms of the remaining three criteria, but I now real-ized that the obvious criterion that led many people to distinguish Gearhart's and Thomson's research was not necessarily violated by ES cell research.

On further reflection, I became confident that, at least for the foreseeable future, researchers using ES cell lines would not have to violate the other three criteria, either. They would neither be directly encouraging others to destroy embryos nor promoting the wider acceptance of or conferring legit-imacy on embryo destruction. Key to understanding this is a fact that had become salient for me during my work in the area of infertility medicine. Embryo destruction on a large scale is now an inseparable part of reproduc-tive medicine. All over the world couples using IVF routinely produce more embryos than they can transfer to the womb. The remaining viable embryos are usually frozen and stored, but most are never used and are eventually discarded. In Britain regulations established by the Human Fertilisation and Embryology Authority (HFEA) require that embryos not used within five years be destroyed unless the progenitors request that they be retained. In 1996 more than 3000 spare embryos, about half those in storage, were de-stroyed as a result of these regulations.[324] Remarkably, the progenitors of about 650 of these embryos never even responded to HFEA inquiries about what should be done with them. In the United States no national legislation exists on this matter. Couples and infertility clinics usually together determine what will be done with the spare embryos. Because of this, it is difficult to know how many embryos are routinely destroyed, but one can suppose the number is large. Until the distant future time when IVF becomes so efficient that it is possible reliably to produce a pregnancy with a single embryo, thousands of spare embryos will be produced by infertility medicine. Only a relative few of these will be needed to produce immortalized pluripotent stem cell lines for research.

This background makes it reasonable to affirm that future researchers using ES cell lines produced from spare embryos need not violate any of the criteria that identify morally culpable cooperation with evil. These researchers will not themselves be involved in the destruction of embryos (that would nevertheless continue in infertility clinics as part of their legal or contractual duties). Assuming that neither the progenitors nor the infertility clinics were paid for these embryos or cell lines (above and beyond the costs of providing them) no financial encouragement by ES cell researchers to destroy them would be involved. Would the prospect of research benefits lead to wider acceptance of this destruction or otherwise endorse, confer legitimacy on, or dilute the condemnation of it? In answering this question, it helps to bear in mind the fact that most progenitors who currently choose to discard spare embryos do so for reasons having nothing to do with the prospect of research (e.g., they have decided to end their parenting quest, they are unwilling to donate spare embryos to other couples, they no longer wish to pay the costs of cryopreservation, etc.). Because many of these people urgently wish to start a family, they are usually unwilling to release spare embryos until they have definitively resolved their infertility problem one way or the other. This suggests that little likelihood exists at the beginning of this process, no matter what the promise of ES cell research, that couples will actually produce embryos for research purposes. Only those embryos that they have otherwise decided to discard at the end of this process will become available for research. In sum, it is unlikely that the research benefits of ES cell research will have much of an impact on the widespread current practices of embryo destruction. One may object to these practices, but ES cell research has little bearing on them.

The insight that, once we get beyond the misleading example provided by James Thomson's initial work, ES and EG cell research are morally very similar has significant implications. It lends ethical substance to the legal position the NIH was trying to develop. As I indicated, the idea that the government could fund research that utilizes ES cells without being morally involved in the derivation of the cell lines seemed at first ridiculous. The government knows where these lines come from and what is being done to produce them. It may even be reimbursing cooperating infertility clinics for the bare costs of producing cell lines from existing frozen embryos. How can it not be complicitous with these deeds? Ordinarily in law and ethics one is not absolved from responsibility for wrongful deeds if one knowingly employs an agent to perform them.[325] Would not the NIH be doing just that if it requested ES cell lines from infertility clinicians? Nevertheless, when we realize that embryos are routinely destroyed and that this tissue would otherwise be washed down a drain or incinerated, its use by government-funded researchers becomes far less problematic. Infertility clinicians who are destroying embryos are not "agents" of the NIH or the downstream researchers. They are performing a task requested of them by the embryos' progenitors or required by clinic or other regulations. On closer examination, this is a case not of the government turning a blind eye while others "do its dirty work," but of funded researchers deriving some benefit from practices over which they have no control.

The insight that research based on ES cell lines does not constitute a culpable instance of cooperation with evil was also important in terms of the prospects for moral consensus both in our working group and in society at large. In the course of thinking about this issue, I sometimes tested my reasoning by asking the following question: "Could a devout Roman Catholic scientist who believes that life begins at conception do research using established pluripotent stem cell lines?" Working through the criteria Bob Wachbroit had provided suggested an affirmative answer. This conclusion was reinforced when I looked more closely at some existing Roman Catholic discussions of the issue of "cooperation with evil."

Most of these discussions are found in older moral treatises and catechetical manuals and focus on such specialized questions as whether a Roman Catholic wife can licitly engage in sex with a husband who resorts to coitus interruptus (she can).[326] But several contemporary discussions of the issue are found in a volume produced by a Roman Catholic biomedical center during the late 1980s in response to the fetal transplantation issue.[327] The most focused of these discussions drew on prior doctrinal treatments of the issue of cooperation.[328] Its author, Russell Smith, contended that it would be unethical for Catholic researchers or tissue recipients to use materials derived from deliberately aborted fetuses. What is noteworthy about his discussion, however, is the acknowledged absence of clear-cut support for this conclusion. Smith observes that such use of fetal tissue would not directly violate any Roman Catholic norm prohibiting the intentional performance of wrongful acts or assistance in them. The wrongfulness, if any, of using fetal tissue for him rests narrowly on the possibility of "scandal." This is a classic Roman Catholic concept used to describe those acts (such as merely being present during idolatrous religious services) that are not wrong in themselves but that ought to be avoided because, through misinterpretation, they "provide occasion for" or run the risk of inciting others to wrongful acts. Of course, impressionable people can misinterpret virtually any act, and we would miss out on many positive things if we tried to avoid all possibility of scandal. As a result, the determination of whether a particular act involves an unacceptable degree of scandal requires a balancing of the benefits of performing the act against the evils it might incite. Other Roman Catholic treatments of scandal warn against being dissuaded from performing clearly beneficial acts merely because of these risks. One source states flatly that "it would not be right, for the sake of avoiding scandal, to inflict serious harm or loss on oneself or the community."[329]

These discussions led me to believe that some individuals standing fully within the Roman Catholic moral tradition could justify beneficial research using human ES cell lines. Some whose consciences were troubled by even a remote degree of involvement in what they regarded as evil might conclude otherwise. But reflection on this issue would be highly individualized and would not separate Roman Catholics as a group from non-Roman Catholics. Some conscientious and well-informed Catholics could be found on both sides of the issue. Formal Roman Catholic thinking on this issue also paralleled moral reasoning generally. The discussions of "cooperation" in this tradition pointed in much the same direction as did our four criteria. This suggested to me that individuals strongly opposed to embryo destruction might come to diverse conclusions about the acceptability of *using* ES cell lines. Many, regardless of their religious views or valuation of embryonic life, would find the use of ES cell lines permissible. Here was the possibility of the common ground we were seeking.

Before I could feel confident about this conclusion, however, one other conceptual hurdle had to be surmounted. There seemed to be one additional feature of ES cell research that distinguished it from Gearhart's EG research and that might provoke concern. In order to produce an ES cell line, it is necessary to remove the inner cell mass from a living embryo. This dissection terminates the embryo's possibility for continued development into a human individual. A telephone call to Brigid Hogan confirmed my suspicion that it was not currently possible to remove just some of these cells, leaving the embryo intact and able to develop. Hence, the preparation of an ES cell line brought together in one act the killing of the embryo and its dissection for research purposes. EG cell research, in contrast, completely separated the act of killing (abortion) from tissue preparation.

Is this difference morally significant? Does this difference in the derivation of the tissues somehow make downstream users of ES cell lines more complicitous in the "evil" acts? These questions are acute for those who view the embryo as a fully protectable being but who want to permit at least the use of tissues derived from its destruction. The argument could be made that, apart from its possible research use, the embryo would not be dissected. Hence, downstream researchers are at least encouraging a type of behavior—"the dissection for research purposes of a living human being"—that would not otherwise occur. This seems to violate Wachbroit's second criterion, which identifies as blameworthy those actions involving direct encouragement to evil.

But what really is the evil at issue here? Research or no research, the embryo will be destroyed.[330] This means it will be thawed and eventually incinerated or otherwise discarded. British infertility clinics, in the course of performing their legally mandated duty of discarding 3300 unwanted or unclaimed embryos, are reported to have thawed and administered a few drops of alcohol to each embryo before incinerating them.[331] It would seem that even for those who oppose embryo destruction, the morally relevant conduct here is the destruction, not how it is accomplished. Once one has set about destroying an early embryo, it seems immaterial whether this is done by thawing and allowing it to die in a petri dish, by dropping it into a lethal solution, or by using a micropipette to disaggregate it. No one denies that early embryos lack sensory organs or tissues. They cannot suffer pain. Their moral worth, if any, resides in their potential for further development. The "wrong" here (if there is any wrong at all) is the ending of that potential, not *how* it is ended. Downstream researchers may thus be involved in encouraging clinicians and others to adopt a particular *method* of embryo destruction, but that is morally unimportant. They are in no way involved in encouraging the destruction itself, which will occur in any case. On a reasonable construal of these acts, downstream researchers would merely be encouraging adoption of a morally neutral method that is most likely to produce some benefit from an otherwise unavoidable situation of loss.

Working through these thoughts, I had no illusions that this approach would end the controversy over ES cell research. Some people would continue to abhor even the most remote connection with what they regarded as evil deeds. Others would see symbolic issues within these debates that threatened the sanctity of human life. They would see the involvement of researchers in the killing of a form of human life as a dangerous precedent that outweighed the benefits of ES cell research. Though I appreciated these concerns, I did not see them as outweighing the possible benefits of ES cell research. I believed that many people who hold a different view of the early embryo's status than I could share my conclusions about using embryos that would otherwise be destroyed. My aim was to develop a position that could attract enough support from a middle ground to shape public policy. The challenge was to understand the issues sufficiently to determine which analogies, precedents, or illustrations best conveyed their underlying logic. Once that determination was made, one could identify those arguments most likely to convey the issues honestly and effectively to a larger audience. Simultaneously, one could better understand the force of one's opponents' views and how to respond to them. The image of researchers dissecting tiny human beings should not be allowed to dominate the discussion. The public had to understand that the key issue was whether spare embryos would be used for valuable research that could save human lives or would merely be thrown away. This was not a matter of countering one emotionally evocative image with another. Rather, it was an attempt to articulate the real nature of the choices and their most likely moral implications.

With these thoughts in place, I spent the weeks and months of late spring and summer finalizing drafts of our subgroup's treatment of the ethical issues involved in the stem cell debate. At Audrey Chapman's request, I took the lead in putting these drafts together in a coherent document, which required revising major portions of the draft by the religious and spiritual subgroup to enhance its consistency with our ethical conclusions. Throughout this process, my experience on the Human Embryo Research Panel weighed heavily on my mind. I believed that Congress was not yet ready to reverse its position on human embryo research. This meant that research involving the derivation of ES cell lines would not be permitted. The NIH was right to try to craft a position that allowed government-funded researchers to use established pluripotent stem cell lines. Congressional and other opponents would probably challenge that position in the courts. But the NIH had a good chance of winning the argument. The law prohibited only research "in which" embryos are destroyed. The members of Congress who had written to Donna Shalala maintained that this prohibition included research that "depended on" the destruction of embryos. But this interpretation was strained and raised major legal issues. If it was accepted, it threatened to extend numerous existing legal prohibitions to the whole range of their antecedent conditions. No judge would want to open that door.

On the political front, small signs began to appear that, where promising directions in biomedical studies related to embryo research and reproductive medicine were concerned, many in Congress had begun to tire of the obstructionist efforts of the anti-abortion lobby. The pharmaceutical and biomedical lobby had already effectively blocked a series of hasty efforts to ban cloning research. When Harold Varmus testified in support of federally funded pluripotent stem cell research in January 1999, members of Congress from all sides of the political spectrum warmly greeted him. Later in the year, Republican senators, including Arlen Specter and Strom Thurmond, came out in support of ES cell research, and Specter introduced a bill to fund it.[332] (Thurmond's daughter suffers from juvenile diabetes.) This suggests that in the minds of at least some people opposed to abortion, the needs of health care research were growing in importance. Given this slow shift in attitudes— a shift, I think, caused by an emerging science-driven perception of the value of some embryo-related research—it was doubtful that the congressional opponents of ES cell research could pass a new law banning the use of these cells. At the same time, it was unlikely that the older prohibition on embryo research would be repealed. Hence, anything that supported the NIH's proposed distinction between use and derivation favored a judicial settlement of the issues and enhanced the chances that this research would begin under federal auspices. In the future, if pluripotent stem cell research proved its value, as fetal tissue transplantation research had begun to do, a broader review of embryo research generally by Congress might be possible.

As our working group moved forward in these directions, NBAC was taking an entirely different course. Late in June, while working on its own report, the commission took a straw vote that recommended that Congress make an exception to the current ban on human embryo research. This exception would permit government-funded researchers both to derive and use ES cell lines. Apparently, several influential members of the commission, including the lawyer and bioethicist Alex Capron, were not persuaded by the use-versus-derivation distinction. A *New York Times* story quoted Capron as saying, "We ought not hide behind the idea that this is just use. That is what the N.I.H. tried to do, but I don't think it will convince the people who need to be convinced."[333] The same story reported that Tom Murray, my colleague from the Human Embryo Research Panel, thought differently. Asking his colleagues whether NBAC might not better retain the use-versus-derivation distinction, Murray said, "I think we speak to a great number of Americans who have complex views and who are undecided, and many of these will find a distinction between use and derivation useful with respect to public funding." The majority of the commissioners chose not to agree with Tom.

I understood what was motivating him. Having watched Congress eviscerate the recommendations of the embryo panel, I knew there was little chance that a substantially unchanged House would permit the exception for which NBAC was asking. To argue that use and derivation were inseparable would also invite the conclusion that the only feasible course of action was to ban both. For NBAC to take this position would undermine the NIH's efforts to find a way to initiate government funding and oversight in this crucial research area.[334] On all these counts, political realism supported both Murray's arguments as well as the position the AAAS group was developing.

But this was not simply a matter of political realism. The use-versus-derivation distinction, I believe, is *morally* valid. It grows out of two important moral considerations. One is the issue of involvement in evil itself. We must be able to draw some line between wrongful actions and the beneficial results that can sometimes be traced back to them. It is not the case that a benefit must be rejected merely because it depends on some preceding evil. If this were so, all the cultural creations built on the backs of forced labor, from the pyramids to Monticello, would have to be leveled. Thinking this issue through honestly and conscientiously is morally crucial and should not be rejected out of hand as casuistical nonsense. As difficult as it is for me to accept, I know that even the Holocaust might offer up some instances that illuminate this fact: it is sometimes better to live with the fruits of wickedness than to reject or destroy them. Finding a better way to honor the dead than by removing an anatomy textbook from the shelves is one example.

A second moral consideration that recommends the use-versus-derivation distinction concerns civic responsibility in a pluralistic democracy. I am convinced that religious groups act unjustly and disrespectfully when they impose their particular and non-publicly shared moral beliefs on others. By *non-publicly shared* I mean those beliefs that derive from special religious premises and that cannot otherwise be supported through evidence and arguments based on common sense or factual claims that reasonably commend themselves to other people.[335] Some religious groups have acted unjustly in the area of embryo research by subordinating considerations of public health to such non-publicly shared beliefs. I develop this point further in the conclusion of this book. Likewise, if religious minorities have a civic duty to put aside their special concerns out of respect for other individuals and for the common good, governments and other citizens have a complementary obligation to respect the sensibilities of religious minorities so long as this can be done without significantly threatening the common good. Amy Gutmann and Dennis Thompson express this idea when they argue for a principle of "accommodation" in the making of public policy. This principle "calls on citizens to try to minimize the range of their public disagreement by promoting policies on which their principles converge, even if they would otherwise place those policies significantly lower on their own list of political priorities."[336] The idea of accommodation finds expression in our constitutional protection of the free exercise of religion and the requirement that religious freedom be overridden only for the most compelling of reasons.

The first of these paired obligations—respect for the common good—tells me that embryo and ES cell research based on cell lines derived from spare embryos must now go forward under public auspices in order adequately to protect the health and welfare of all citizens. The second obligation—respect for the religious views of others—tells me that at each phase of embryo and reproductive research, efforts should be made to avoid unnecessary incursions on some citizens' sensibilities.[337] At this time, these two obligations translate into permission for federally funded use of pluripotent stem cell lines, but not their derivation.[338] A policy based on this distinction is morally as well as politically sound.

I acknowledge that future events may lead me to rethink some of my conclusions. It may be found that some crucially important areas of ES cell research require active involvement of the researcher in the derivation of the cell lines. During a meeting of the AAAS working group in late July, Eric Meslin, the executive director of NBAC, told us that this consideration was one factor that influenced NBAC's position. Eric reported that some scientists had told the commission that work like James Thomson's, in which the researcher was involved in all its phases, would probably mark the early period of ES cell research. This view, which was reiterated at length in the final NBAC report on stem cells,[339] apparently was supported by a number of scientists NBAC consulted. Nevertheless, it directly contradicted the opinion of the scientists in our group. More important, it is not supported by almost two decades of experience with mouse ES cells, in which research on established cell lines predominates. Scientists, of course, usually want maximal liberty to pursue their research. I suspect that NBAC had accredited some of the scientific opinions they heard justifying the importance of cell line derivation partly in order to support a majority of the commissioners' moral discomfort with the use-versus-derivation distinction.[340] If derivation proves to have a high degree of scientific importance, however, it may be necessary to rethink the use-versus-derivation distinction.

Future developments also may erode the emphasis on spare embryos implicit in this distinction. As I have argued, the moral logic of separating use from derivation rests on the fact that the needed embryos can come from the population of those embryos left over from infertility procedures that will otherwise be destroyed. However, we can already imagine a future in which it may be desirable deliberately to create embryos in order to produce autologous pluripotent stem cell lines. This is the prospect I sketched earlier of using a somatic cell from an individual to produce an embryo (via somatic cell nuclear transfer technology), and from this embryo, a histocompatible ES cell line for cell replacement therapy.[341] Before "therapeutic cloning" of this sort becomes a reality, and certainly before it merits federal research support, many questions will have to be asked. Is it really not possible to avoid this alternative by manipulating immunity factors in existing pluripotent stem cell lines produced from spare embryos (research that could be done with federal dollars)? Does the actual bench research in this area need federal support and oversight, or is it something that can be accomplish effectively with private funding? And if this possibility becomes a clinical therapy, will it need federal support, or can it be offered as a purchased clinical service? The answers to these questions are by no means evident. If cell replacement therapies using deliberately created embryos prove highly successful, we may also have to consider issues of federal funding beyond the research context, in the area of clinical services. Would it be just to deny Medicaid or Medicare recipients access to these therapies merely because other citizens morally object to them?

Fortunately, these are questions for the future. I introduce them here to illustrate how ongoing experience can force a rethinking of moral conclusions from one period to the next. This is exactly what happened with fetal tissue transplantation research, support for which has been reinforced by increasing clinical successes and the efficacy of morally sound regulations.

I must stress that there are two things I am *not* saying in indicating the importance of ongoing experience and the possibility of revising our conclusions. First, I am not suggesting that we should advocate the least offensive research initiatives now as a political device for expanding these initiatives later. I am not a political scientist and have no idea whether this is the best way to proceed. I am making a moral, not a political, argument. It is respect for others, not political efficacy, that requires the use of the least offensive means needed at each stage of research. Second, I am not suggesting that success makes something that is wrong right. I personally do not believe that human embryo research, including the deliberate creation of embryos for valid research or clinical purposes, is wrong, but I acknowledge that many people do. I am not saying that the mere fact of scientific or clinical success will convince these people otherwise or prove them wrong. I am saying that moral reasoning must always be in conversation with human experience. Because so many aspects of moral decision require difficult balancing judgments often based on uncertain predictions about future harms or benefits, it is very important to stay in touch with moral realities as they evolve "on the ground." It may be that all the promises of human embryo or pluripotent stem cell research will prove to be fruitless. In that case, the urgency of this research and the justification of continued federal funding for research will decline. Conversely, the clinical successes may be enormous. They may also spur new techniques for producing pluripotent stem cell lines that reduce or minimize the need to destroy embryos. In that case, those currently opposed to these research directions may find themselves altering their opposition to some forms of this research. Remaining open to experience does not mean sacrificing principles to success. It merely expresses the wisdom that as human beings we are not omniscient or unerringly right in our moral judgments.

On 25 August, the AAAS and Institute for Civil Society sponsored a public forum at AAAS headquarters in Washington to present our working group's main findings and recommendations. These were also posted immediately on the AAAS website, with a published version of the report to follow some weeks later.[342] Throughout the morning and early afternoon spokespersons for each of our subgroups offered brief presentations. I gave an overview of the ethical issues and met over lunch with the press. From midafternoon on, I found myself swept back five years in time. The afternoon session, reserved for comments and questions from the public, was reminiscent of so many I had suffered through on the Human Embryo Research Panel. A Washington grapevine apparently exists among anti-abortion groups. As soon as questions and comments were permitted, people lined up at the two microphones to protest ES and EG stem cell research. Among the objectors was my old intellectual nemesis, Richard Doerflinger. I realized from materials I had read that Doerflinger was once again taking the lead in mustering opposition to NIH funding of this research. At the beginning of the year, he had testified before a Senate appropriations subcommittee.[343] Not surprisingly, positions he expressed, as well as some of his exact words, appeared in the letters and statements issued by members of Congress opposed to this research. It is no exaggeration to say that Richard Doerflinger and his office (the Bishops' Secretariat for Pro-life Activities) constitute the most active and effective center of opposition to all facets of human embryo research—and now to both EG and ES cell research as well. During the afternoon, Richard reappeared at the microphone several times. As he had done in his written documents, he challenged the need for and value of ES cell research. He repeatedly asked why success could not be obtained using only adult stem cells. Scientists on our panel replied that adult stem cells had serious limits, that research on *all* cell types was needed to better assess their comparative value, and that reliance on adult cells alone would greatly slow progress.[344] These opinions had already been supported by other leading scientists, including Brigid Hogan in her recent testimony before NBAC.[345] Despite this, Doerflinger here, and in his published writings, continued to insist that adult stem cells should be the sole initial source of research materials.[346] In his world there are no significant opportunity costs to limiting research to a less promising direction.

As the day wore on, several of my colleagues at the table, as well as Audrey Chapman and our working group's usually cheerful assistant, Michele Garfinkle, grew more somber. "Was this the way our recommendations would be met? Is the public really so hostile to ES and EG cell research?," several of them asked. It was my moment, as an old hand, to be upbeat. "Don't measure the country's mood by Washington, D.C., and the people who turn out for these meetings," I said. "We are not seeing a representative audience." Though I knew this to be the case, I also realized that well organized lobbying groups bringing pressure to bear on a small number of pivotal members of Congress exerted far more weight in this area than numbers indicated. The road to federal support for pluripotent stem cell research was filled with obstacles.

In September NBAC issued its final report. As the earlier straw vote had indicated, the commission chose to dismiss the use-versus-derivation distinction and to recommend federal funding for ES cell research in its entirety. The final report draws heavily on the position developed by Ronald Dworkin in his book *Life's Dominion*.[347] There, Dworkin argues that, despite their obvious disagreements, those opposed to abortion and those who favor choice share a commitment to the sanctity and intrinsic value of human life.[348] This element of agreement, Dworkin maintains, is reflected in the relative consensus on the legitimacy of abortion when a woman's life and health are imperiled. Applying this argument to the stem cell issue, the NBAC report held that a similar consensus on the sanctity of human life legitimates ES cell research involving both the derivation and use of cell lines. Despite differing estimates of the value of the early human embryo, the report maintains, many people can agree that early human embryos may be destroyed when this research promises new lifesaving medical therapies.[349] The report applies this reasoning to spare embryos only. Apart from some expressions of concern about the "instrumentalization of human life," the NBAC report does not explain why its Dworkin-based reasoning does not also apply to the deliberate creation of embryos for these beneficial purposes.

Unfortunately, even when restricted to spare embryos, this whole line of argument is unconvincing, both in Dworkin's book and in NBAC's application of it. First, it is simply untrue that many that oppose abortion and embryo research would permit the killing of embryos or fetuses to save other human lives through medical research. The formal Roman Catholic position on this issue is that one may never directly and intentionally kill an innocent human being (a category to which Roman Catholic thought assigns the embryo and fetus), even to save another person's life. Quite consistently with this position, Roman Catholic teaching prohibits abortion when a pregnancy threatens the mother's life, even if this means that both mother and child die as a result. Apart from this particular feature of Roman Catholic thought, the belief that members of anti-abortion and anti-embryo research groups would permit the killing of embryos or fetuses to create medical cures is, quite simply, a misjudgment of that entire movement. This is precisely the hierarchy of values that they reject. In the course of our 25 August forum, several individuals suffering from life-threatening diseases like Type I diabetes spoke out against ES cell research. They would rather suffer the terrible consequences of their disorder, they said, than be a party to what they regard as morally evil research.[350] NBAC's reasoning for its position is not only unlikely to reach these people, but it badly misrepresents their priorities. Although it is true that some or many opponents of abortion would permit abortion when a pregnant woman's life is endangered, this exception clearly does not extend to the destruction of embryos for the purpose of lifesaving medical research. If it did, little or no resistance would be raised to embryo research.

By now, it should be clear that I am uncomfortable with the way in which NBAC has chosen to approach human embryo research and, to some extent, public bioethics as a whole. Sometimes, I believe, it has overly politicized the advisory process by paying too much attention to what its members perceive as political currents and concerns. This is reflected in its haste to address the cloning issue, its privileging of religious views, and its reluctance even to raise the issue of embryo research in the cloning context in which it was highly important to do so. NBAC paid a price for this failure to address the issue of embryo research when pluripotent stem cell research made it impossible to avoid it any longer. Even then, its resulting position suggested an unwillingness to confront society's deep divisions on this issue and openly defend a moral position against its critics. Doing so would require a direct confrontation with unacceptable alternative positions and clear arguments as to why these alternatives should not dictate public policy. NBAC did nothing like this. Forced by the pace of science to reconsider embryo research, it sought to justify its position by appealing to a nonexistent consensus.

A deeper problem is the lack of penetrating moral analysis in some of NBAC's thinking. No one expects a bioethics commission or expert panel to inflict philosophical treatises on the public. However, these groups are considered expert because their members are able to arrive at a penetrating understanding of the basic issues and choices. This is no less true of the ethicists on a panel than it is of its scientists and lawyers. On the basis of this understanding, the panel must build clear and convincing public arguments to convey the gist of its conclusions. I believe that the Human Embryo Research Panel tried to do just this. My evidence for this assertion is that years after its publication, the panel's report remains a key reference for all those concerned with public funding for embryo research, from Geron's Ethics Advisory Board to NBAC itself. I believe that the public is not served by arguments that misrepresent existing positions or that hastily dismiss options, such as the use-versus-derivation distinction, that merit closer attention.

This tendency to avoid incisive analysis is particularly evident in the NBAC report's treatment of the use-versus-derivation distinction. Having apparently concluded that the distinction might strike some members of the public as facile, the commission rejected it and called for an exception to the current ban on federally funded embryo research in order to permit both the use and derivation of stem cell lines.[351] In seeking to justify its position, the NBAC report mentions several scientific and legal considerations that seem less like compelling arguments than matters advanced to support a previously arrived at moral conclusion.[352] On the surface, this moral commitment to use and derivation might seem commendable in terms of its willingness to challenge the current legal prohibition on funding for embryo research. However, the net effect of this stance was to put forward a politically ill-fated recommendation that simultaneously undermined the position the NIH was trying to defend—all for no good moral reason. The use-versus-derivation distinction is morally tenable. The course of genuine moral boldness would have been to develop arguments that could make this clear, not to retreat before feared objections.

A similar lack of penetrating analysis marks NBAC's handling of the issue of research embryos in connection with ES cell research. This possibility will certainly grow in importance as researchers try to develop means of producing autologous stem cell lines for tissue repair. Such cell lines require the deliberate creation of embryos that will not be transferred to a womb. Shortly after publishing his first report on EG stem cell research, John Gearhart, writing with a coauthor, stressed the importance of this issue by stating that "society must decide whether the therapeutic benefits justify denying full development to the constructed embryos."[353] Nevertheless, despite the imminence of these choices, NBAC chose to avoid the issue. Although it allowed that the ban on research embryos might have to be reconsidered in light of future developments,[354] the report offered little analysis of the issues and recommended limiting research now to the use of spare embryos only.[355] The principal concern mentioned was the familiar, but vague, worry about the "instrumentalization" of human life. What the report fails to address, however, is why the creation of embryos for lifesaving research raises the question of instrumentalization, while a couple's knowing creation of many more embryos than they need for reproductive purposes does not. Because most initial research can be done with spare embryos, the report's recommendation that research begin using only spare embryos was a reasonable one, but the commission's failure to provide a thorough examination of the issues is troubling. By effectively ratifying the distinction between research and spare embryos without providing countervailing arguments, the commission created a problem for itself in the event that future research demonstrates the value and need for federal funding of research on created embryos.

Some believe that NBAC's reticence was wise. In a paper prepared for NBAC's deliberations on the stem cell issue, the bioethicist John C. Fletcher urged the commission to defer consideration of the issue of creating autologous stem cell lines through cloning or other means. Defending his view, Fletcher approvingly quotes a statement made in 1984 by Britain's Council for Science and Society. Those involved in ethical debates on new technologies, said the council, should "refrain from moral judgment on unverifiable possibilities."[356] But the development of autologous stem cell lines is hardly an unverifiable possibility; it is the therapeutic goal of stem cell research and is already being pursued by leading companies like Geron and Advanced Cell Technology. Fletcher also lists among the primary responsibilities of an expert commission the need to "educate the public on the nature, promise, and risks of pluripotential stem cell (PSC) research."[357] This is just what NBAC failed to do. Seeking to bypass an ethically and politically controversial issue, NBAC missed the chance to advance public understanding of an impending area for decision.

As I write in January 2001, the stem cell issue remains unresolved. On 3 December 1999 the NIH issued its proposed guidelines for federally funded human pluripotent stem cell research.[358] These continued to affirm the use-versus-derivation distinction and amplified the research protections afforded to donors of embryonic tissue. Following an extended period of public comment, a final set of guidelines was issued on August 25, 2000.[359] At least one Senate bill is pending that would permit federal funding of research involving the derivation and use of stem cell lines from spare embryos,[360] but at least twenty senators have already announced their opposition to the initiative.[361]

Late on a Friday afternoon in October 1999, I received an e-mail message from The Patient's Cure, a lobbying organization that seeks to promote federal support for research on a host of disease conditions. "Would you be willing to meet with the editorial board of The Washington Post to help persuade them to urge Congress to support stem cell research?" I agreed do so, and on Monday I found myself with a small group of scientists and patients' advocates gathered in a conference room. The actual meeting was somewhat disappointing to me. Amy Schwartz, the lead writer on the issue, seemed more interested in scientific information than moral reasoning. As we left the building, I recall feeling that I had been unable to convey the message I wanted. Nevertheless, to my surprise, several days later The Washington Post published a lead editorial with the headline "Miracle Cells." Stating that it "was reasonable for Congress not to let public funds go directly to the destruction of human embryos," the editorial nevertheless favored the NIH's position that the agency should use, but not derive, ES cells. It continued by saying that, when it comes to research "where the embryos used were being destroyed anyway, . . . the rationale for blocking an explosively promising field falls apart."[362]

Although The Washington Post represents a liberal editorial position, it seldom gets too far ahead of the congressional mainstream. Witness the devastating impact of its editorial five years before on the Human Embryo Research Panel's recommendation for research embryos. Now its caution led it to support public funding for ES cell research using, but not deriving, spare embryos. This was essentially a summary of the AAAS position I had defended at the editorial meeting. This time the Post was not an adversary, but a friend. Obviously, I had learned from past experience to stress what was minimally required to expedite a needed research direction. Thinking back to the experience of the Human Embryo Research Panel, I continue to wonder whether less stress on research embryos and more on the use of the spare embryos that were otherwise going to waste might have hastened our work as well as the acceptance of our report. But I was not alone in changing over time. The science surrounding human embryo research had predictably moved forward. The stakes for everyone, and not only the community of infertile people, were becoming clear. The *Post*'s enthusiastic support of stem cell research and acceptance of my arguments was a sign of all these changes. Has Congress also changed? Will it now authorize some ES cell research? Will it at least permit the NIH to move unchallenged in this direction? As I write, the debate is once again about to begin.

CONCLUSION

A FEW years ago, I was invited to speak in a course organized by a woman I had known for several years. Beth was in her late thirties. Like many other women of her generation, she had delayed marriage and child-bearing in order to start her career. The last time we met, two years before, she was thrilled to tell me that she was pregnant. Now, as we talked, I could see that her elation was gone. That first pregnancy, she reported, had ended in a miscarriage after several weeks. Since then, there had been two more very early miscarriages. She and her husband were in the first phase of an extensive medical work-up to determine what was wrong. Her physicians talked of immune system problems and her body's reactions to the foreign tissues of an embryo. They were urging an experimental therapy to prompt her immune system to react appropriately. As Beth recounted this to me, I looked at her face. Around her eyes were lines of fatigue and pain. Although she insisted that she and her husband were not infertile—after all, they could conceive a child—it was clear to me that they had entered the difficult world of reproductive medicine.

It is because of people like Beth and her husband that I first became involved in the ethics of assisted reproduction and human embryo research. Every day, thousands of people in the United States and elsewhere struggle with infertility and failed pregnancies. Their physical and emotional suffering

165

is frequently downplayed or ignored. This attitude of neglect is reflected in the absence of sufficient federal support for research in the area of human reproductive medicine and the existing ban on support for human embryo research. This deliberate and sustained withholding of federal dollars from an important research area has no parallel in our history. Although special interests have often steered federal research dollars toward their favored disease condition, no other major research area has been systematically starved of funds as a result of political intervention.

What began as a hardship for a subpopulation of infertile people now affects us all through its negative impact on stem cell research. If this research is slowed because of a lack of federal support, thousands of individuals in the decades ahead will suffer or die needlessly from diabetes, heart disease, and many other disorders that cell replacement therapies could cure. This confirms the insight that research freedom is a seamless garment. One cannot label a vital research area "off limits" or declare it ineligible for federal support without impeding the pursuit of knowledge generally. An involvement in this area that began for me with people like Beth is now motivated by the awareness that ill-guided prohibitions imperil the advance of U.S. biomedical research in general.

One reason for this record of research obstruction is the widespread public indifference to the problems of the infertile. As I indicated in the first chapter, for most people infertility is a distant and poorly understood concern. Another reason, as we can now see, is the difficulty of some of the underlying ethical issues. Research at the beginnings of life raises new questions and imposes new choices. Where should we draw lines on the continuum of nascent human life? How do we balance attention to concerns about the sanctity of human life against the need to protect and promote human health? What are our obligations to the unconceived or the unborn, and how do we balance these obligations against what is owed to their parents? Throughout this book, I have tried to offer new ways of thinking about these questions. I have also tried to indicate why I believe that the needs of children and adults take priority over the moral claims of human life in its earliest forms. This belief alone justifies human embryo research.

Unfortunately, another troublesome ethical question must be considered, one that is probably more relevant to understanding this history of research obstruction. This is the question of whether religious groups are justified, solely on the basis of their theological and religious views, in seeking to control the direction of federally funded biomedical research. This question is important because the organized opposition to federal support in this area has been marshaled largely by religious groups committed to the view that the early embryo is a research subject meriting all the protections afforded children. Although some people who oppose specific forms of embryo research, such as cloning or the use of research embryos, accept the right of abortion, the most vehement opponents of embryo research generally tend to stand within the religiously affiliated anti-abortion movement.

My experiences on the Human Embryo Research Panel and the AAAS working group confirm this observation. Most of those who appeared before us to speak against embryo research were members of religious groups or organizations opposed to abortion. The Roman Catholic Church's presence, embodied in the person of Richard Doerflinger, was most evident. Also very prominent was the American Life League. This group, which identifies itself as "the largest grass-roots, pro-life educational organization in the United States," bases its stands on Roman Catholic teachings.[363] Conservative Protestants and some Orthodox Jews also entered into the debate, either individually or through religiously affiliated pro-life organizations. In the minds of these opponents, embryo research is an assault on the sanctity of human life. They regard the early embryo as morally equivalent to any other child or adult human subject and believe that it should not be involved in research that exposes it to risks of injury or death unless these risks are directly related to efforts to increase its chances of survival. For many of these people, it is irrelevant that the embryo may otherwise be doomed, as is true of the many frozen spare embryos remaining from infertility procedures that will eventually be thawed and discarded.[364] They view these embryos as dying persons who may not be subjected to harmful procedures without their consent. Proxy consent by the embryos' progenitors is unacceptable because these progenitors are not regarded as having the embryos' best interests at heart. Recently, a powerful lobbying effort based on this reasoning has tried to halt NIH funding of ES stem cell research.[365]

It is not difficult to see that this position on the status of the early embryo cannot legally or ethically be a basis for prohibiting *privately* financed embryo research in this country. Under U.S. law, the early embryo is not a juridical person. It is considered to be bodily tissue under the control of its progenitors. If a woman or couple wished to donate gametes or embryos for the purposes of embryo research, there would be major constitutional obstacles to preventing them from doing so, as some lower court rulings have already implied.[366] I believe that these legal conclusions are ethically correct. It is unreasonable to believe that the claims of the early embryo outweigh those of its parent-progenitors or the health and safety of children and adult women. This leads to the conclusion that infertile couples who wish to donate embryos for research that is aimed at improving the safety and efficacy of procedures in which they are involved or for other biomedical research purposes should have the right to do so. Individuals or couples with a different view of the moral status of the embryo should be permitted to withhold their own embryos from such research. The institution of procedures to secure informed consent should protect these people from coercion or misinformation. Those who are potential recipients of tissues or cells derived from embryos probably also have a right to know the source of the materials being used. This would permit them to choose whether or not to undergo the therapy. But such persons have no right to prohibit others from donating their embryos for these purposes, to limit the ability of privately financed scientific researchers to pursue these areas of investigation, or to prohibit others from benefiting from transplantation research. This means that legal efforts to ban privately funded embryo research are unjust and constitute a violation of public ethical responsibility in a pluralistic democracy.

This leaves for ethical analysis only the very complex issue of *federal funding* of embryo research. As I have indicated throughout this book, the consequences of prohibiting this funding are serious. To a large extent, the slowed progress of infertility medicine and the host of health problems associated with it—including the epidemic of high-order multiple births—stem from the absence of federal funding. With more than 350 infertility programs, the United States is now the world's leading provider and consumer of infertility services. The disproportion between the extent of clinical services and the amount of research being conducted is ethically unacceptable. It is irresponsible for a modern society to permit the widespread provision of medical services without simultaneously fostering the research needed to establish the efficacy and safety of those services. In addition, a pluralistic democracy committed to protecting and improving the health of its citizens cannot justly deny one area research support merely because some of its citizens object to that research on the basis of their personal religious and moral beliefs. Unless objections can be grounded in concerns appropriate to a pluralistic democracy—and this means reasonably clear issues of public health and safety— they must be set aside.

I realize that this position is not self-evident, so I will defend it. First, I think we can dismiss as untenable the view that no citizen should have to pay taxes for governmentally approved and funded research activities to which she or he morally objects. This position, repeatedly articulated by presenters before the Human Embryo Research Panel who objected to embryo research, makes no sense ethically or legally. In an ideal society it might be possible to allow citizens to direct their tax monies to legislated programs they support and away from programs they oppose. In practice, however, this approach would be a nightmare to administer and might effectively give powerful minorities a veto over approved spending programs. Like it or not, paying for legislated programs about which one has ethical reservations is one consequence of living in a democracy. For example, those who oppose U.S. military institutions are not exempted from paying taxes for them, and those who favor private schooling are not permitted to withhold taxes from public schools.

Far more serious is the view that setting priorities among federally funded health research programs should be a matter of majority decision. This, I take it, is the position of those who believe that Congress has acted justly in banning NIH funding of human embryo research. Those who hold this view tend to regard health research as a discretionary social expenditure, like public support for parks, museums, or the arts. Citizens are not wronged if such discretionary funds are steered in directions other than the ones they prefer. No fundamental rights of citizens are involved. Instead, these are properly matters of majority determination. For those who hold this view, issues of scientific merit or a research area's likely contribution to public health take a back seat to voters' preferences. In addition, provided that public funds are not spent on specifically sectarian projects, nothing is wrong if the majority's preferences happen to be shaped by strongly held religious and moral views. Concerning purely discretionary expenditures, all sorts of factors, from aesthetic preferences to religious beliefs, can play a role in shaping public policy. It is also not inappropriate for powerful religious minorities to exert a disproportionate impact on the legislative process, because, once again, only discretionary matters are involved. Indeed, in some people's view, the presence of strong religious disagreements about matters of public policy provides a good reason for the withdrawal of federal funding from a research area.[367]

I believe that this position is wrong and cannot be justified. The core mistake is classifying federally funded health-related research as discretionary and unrelated to the fundamental rights of citizens. Quite the opposite is true. Health-related research today is often a matter of life and death. In a just society, its direction and governance can be of the highest importance, in some cases on a par with other matters bearing on basic constitutional liberties.[368] Thus, research cannot simply become a matter of majority whim or minority pressure. Once the government makes the decision to fund health-related research generally, it is obligated to consider the impact of that research on everyone's health. This requires the allocation of resources equitably, without unjust discrimination among classes of citizens. Policy determinations should be made in terms of publicly defensible scientific and health considerations. This includes the use of independent panels for peer review of the science involved and other multidisciplinary panels for assisting in policy decisions based on the merit and worth of particular research directions. Public opinion and pressure group tactics can play a role in this process by alerting policy makers to the meaning and impact of disease conditions. This is especially important when majority opinion has obscured or misrepresented vital health care needs. But public opinion must always be filtered through a process of objective assessment and peer review.

Specific religious or moral beliefs not grounded in publicly defensible values cannot be allowed to dominate this process. Those involved in the policy determination process must proceed on the basis of what John Rawls has called "liberal political values."[369] They must use arguments grounded in basic and widely shared values and avoid appeal to religiously defined goals or other values that are not widely shared. Among widely shared values are those necessary for the pursuit of human ends generally. They include such things as protection from physical harms, liberty to pursue one's ends (including religious ends consistent with other values), and access to at least a minimum of the material goods and services needed to be a participating member of the social order. Inquiry about and discussion of values and appropriate policies must also be guided by what Rawls has called "public reason." This relies on common sense, reasonableness, and, where appropriate, the use of scientific information and methods, when these are not themselves controversial. Religious beliefs and moral priorities that cannot sustain themselves in these terms should not enter into these discussions. The requirement that policy determination be independent of particular religious, theological, or philosophical beliefs does not mean that people's positions on issues may not be deeply informed by such beliefs. However, once public discussion of policies begins, these beliefs must be capable of being articulated in terms of widely shared liberal political values and the method of "public reason."

The AIDS epidemic offers a good illustration of the position I am trying to convey. During the early phases of the epidemic, many citizens were relatively indifferent to the terrible suffering being experienced by some gay people. Others agreed with the handful of outspoken fundamentalist religious leaders who described AIDS as a divine punishment for sins. Imagine if these attitudes had prevailed. Until its causes are understood and means of controlling it are developed, a novel infectious disease like AIDS represents a threat to everyone's health. Basing policy on non-publicly sustainable religious ideas and neglecting clear facts of disease transmission would have imperiled us all. Beyond this larger threat, if AIDS research had continued to languish, gay citizens would have been justified in believing they had been deprived of the fundamental due process protections of the Constitution. While billions of dollars were being spent annually on cancer and heart disease, the government was neglecting a fatal disease that threatened their lives. In order to put a stop to this injustice, AIDS activists made their presence known on the national scene, sometimes organizing boisterous demonstrations at FDA and NIH headquarters.[370] This history should not be construed as justifying the primacy of political influences in the health research policy process. Just the opposite is true. Political protests represented a minority's assertion of its fundamental right to a share of health-related research in the face of unjust majoritarian indifference and neglect.

Although AIDS represents an especially urgent health concern, the basic lessons of this experience also apply to human embryo research. Currently, whole classes of research related to public health and safety are supported by federal funds. Much of this support is for areas that involve no greater risk to individuals than do either reproductive medicine or the host of disease conditions that can benefit from embryonic stem cell research. Singling out embryo research for a denial of support thus amounts to unjust political intervention in the research prioritizing and funding process. In the area of reproductive medicine, it also amounts to arbitrary discrimination against the women and children affected by poorly researched reproductive medical procedures. Furthermore, this injustice is largely motivated not by reasonable public concerns related to health and safety, but by publicly unsustainable religious and ethical objections.[371]

I realize how difficult it is for many Americans to appreciate these parallels. It is not just that many people are unaware of the health impacts of the lack of federal funding in this area. Many share the religious views that underlie the current ban. They oppose abortion and regard the fetus and embryo as protectable beings. They are strongly opposed to the use of their taxes for what they regard as ethically unacceptable research. Others who do not share these views sometimes support this position, reasoning that the benefits of federal support for human embryo research do not seem to outweigh the direct assault on other citizens' religiously informed ethical sensibilities.

Despite these views, the widespread presence of a particular religious sensibility does not justify its being used as grounds for denying other citizens equal access to the benefits of health-related research. To help in understanding this claim, let me offer an imaginative illustration suggested by the Swiss moral philosopher Alex Mauron.[372] Mauron asks us to think through the social controversy over fetal or embryonic rights by considering the situation of Jain religious believers living in a liberal, pluralistic, and nontheological society. As a matter of deep religious conviction, Jains hold an extreme reverence for life. They are strict vegetarians. Some devout Jains sweep the ground before them while walking to avoid killing small bugs.[373] Imagine, now, that Jains constitute a substantial part of the population of the United States, perhaps even a majority. To what extent should public policy respect their position? For example, would it be just for the government to impose mandatory vegetarianism on all of us by outlawing the slaughter of farm animals? Would it be just to prohibit all use of animals in medical research?

Mauron answers these questions by observing that, although the point of view that Jains represent cannot be summarily dismissed, it should not be made a basis of public policy in a democracy, whether Jains are a minority or a majority. At its foundation, the Jain belief is a religious one informed by a particular metaphysical view of human and animal souls. Without these premises, Jains cannot demonstrate in widely acceptable terms that the killing of animals imposes grave harms on us all. Jains are certainly free to base their own lives and practices on these beliefs. They are also free, Mauron observes, "to try and persuade the rest of us to see things their way." Nevertheless, "they cannot impose their views on non-believers if they want to be peaceful participants in a secular social order."[374] Imposing their beliefs would expose nonbelievers to many serious risks (including exposure to starvation or disease) without their consent and in the absence of reasons that were of compelling validity to everyone. The parallels here to our own public reasoning about abortion are clear. Legal impediments to abortion based on strong views of fetal rights similarly represent the imposition of serious risks on nonbelievers without their consent and in the absence of reasons that are of compelling validity to everyone.[375]

Carrying Mauron's illustration a bit further, imagine that most members of the Jain community have reluctantly agreed to accept the status quo regarding the consumption of meat and animal experimentation. However, some diehard Jain activists remain undeterred. They decide to renew their struggle by concentrating their energies on an emotionally charged sector of biomedical research that uses animals, perhaps primate research. Assume that, on the basis of peer review and careful policy analysis, this research has been found to be vitally necessary for understanding and controlling serious disease conditions. It is also subject to legal and ethical monitoring and permitted only to the extent needed for this purpose. Nevertheless, the Jain activists realize that the public does not understand the purpose or scope of this research very well. They choose to misrepresent it, underplay the consequences of halting it, and argue that it will only lead to the coerced use of human beings in research. Stopping all primate research represents for them an opportunity to slow the killing of animals and to gain a foothold for their moral perspective in national policy.

I can think of four reasons a campaign like this would be morally unacceptable. First, it violates the requirement that in a pluralistic democracy one not use the law to impose one's non-publicly sustainable views on others. Second, it is dishonest. Unable to make a case for animal protection generally, the activists would now be trying to accomplish their goals by means of a "backdoor" approach at a point at which public understanding of the issues is poor. Their use of ostensibly public arguments against a specific form of animal research also masks their basic religious opposition to the killing of any animals. Third, this tactic is discriminatory. The selective elimination of one form of research imposes special harms on people whose health needs depend on it. Finally, this tactic undermines the integrity of an independently established scientific review process.

Analogies, Plato tells us, walk on weak legs. Some will dispute that this imaginative illustration accurately parallels what has transpired in the area of embryo research. I believe, however, that it represents, point for point, a fully accurate description of the basic moral issues and dynamics that have marked this area. That this seems less evident to some people can be traced, I believe, primarily to the two factors I have highlighted. One is the important role that anti-abortion activism continues to play in our public debates about reproductive medicine. The impact of this activism is highlighted by the fact that Great Britain, which has a notably less powerful anti-abortion movement, long ago approved embryo research and, through the Human Fertilisation and Embryology Authority, set up comprehensive national regulations and support for it. A second key factor obscuring understanding of the issue is the absence of public familiarity with the urgent health and safety issues associated with human embryo research. For those lacking this understanding, which I and other members of the Human Embryo Research Panel developed over months of reading and listening, it is easy to dismiss embryo research as a marginal activity related to a marginal and wholly optional area of medical care, infertility medicine. Throughout this book, I have suggested that this dismissal is a serious mistake. The emergence of stem cell research as a major area of contention only points up the risks of continued research obstruction in this area.

Other factors have played a secondary role in this history of research obstruction. One is the widely shared sense of discomfort with scientific intrusions in the heretofore-sacrosanct area of reproduction. This discomfort manifested itself very clearly in public debates over cloning, which inspired even liberal and progressive religious spokespeople to go on record as opposing tampering with the sources of human individuality and the dynamics of human parenting. In the area of embryo research, this broad opposition to manipulating life's beginnings finds expression in the very negative reception given the Human Embryo Research Panel's recommendation that scientists be permitted to deliberately create and use research embryos. This single recommendation was so widely criticized in the press that it led the Clinton White House to back away from it. The opposition continues in the area of pluripotent stem cell research. No public panel, including NBAC or the AAAS working group, has been willing to argue for the legitimacy of deliberately creating embryos as a source of autologous (histocompatible) stem cell lines. In the case of the AAAS working group, this hesitancy was partly founded on the understanding that stem cell research had not yet reached the point at which this was necessary. Nevertheless, the day is not far off when this issue will come to the fore, forcing a reexamination of the widespread resistance to this research.

This debate suggests that concerns about tampering with the sanctity of human life and parenthood do play a contributory role in current efforts to block research in the life sciences, but often these are not the decisive considerations. Rather, the greatest energy for this opposition is drawn from the first two factors I signaled: opposition to anything linked to abortion and public unawareness of the implications of research obstruction.

Those who wish to preserve the freedom of life sciences research in the areas of reproductive medicine and genetics must understand this array of forces. They must increase public understanding of the scientific and medical stakes by improving public education in these areas. They must strive politically and administratively to create a more protected space for expert panels in the policy process. Like other elements of our federal system—for example, the Federal Reserve and the FDA—science research must be insulated from direct and unmediated control by powerful political interest groups. Those wishing to preserve the freedom of life sciences research also must work to counter the often-veiled anti-abortion activism that intrudes on policy processes in these areas, and they must make the public aware of the ethical implications of such intrusions. This requires renewing our understanding of the ethical responsibilities we all share as citizens in a pluralistic democracy. Personal distaste for research in a particular area, however sincerely motivated, must take second place to a reliance on "public reason" in arriving at a common research policy. Imposing our personal views on others' lives and health without resort to widely shared arguments and values is essentially a form of disrespect for fellow citizens. It is a violation of what Rawls calls "the duty of civility."[376] It evidences the notion that the emotional power of one's beliefs and their acceptance by many others is an adequate reason for imposing them on society as a whole.

Finally, we must all resist the temptation to stand pat with older responses to new biological realities. The life sciences are daily changing our understanding of the processes that make us what we are. This does not mean that our basic moral principles are subject to constant scientific revision. Although new biological knowledge is forcing us to rethink our commitment to older boundary lines of moral protection at the beginning and end of life, our ways of thinking about those matters remain the same. In every case, we make a moral decision based on our reasoned and impartial calculus of the benefits and burdens of drawing a line at a particular place. If this approach seems new, it is only because science and technology have forced us to look more closely at what we are doing when we determine where our moral protection begins and ends.

It is the nature of the life sciences today that they will force an understanding of this choice process on us more and more. New choices emerge with almost every new bit of scientific knowledge. Our emerging ability to control the genes that form our bodies gives us new powers to intervene and shape their direction. Not to intervene, although it may often be the wisest choice, is still a choice. Understanding the elaborate programs that unfold from the moment gametes come in contact with one another forces us to make ethical decisions about when and how we may intervene in the ensuing process of development. The position that one sacred moment exists after which all interventions must stop, that "human life begins at conception," reflects not only a single religious ideology, but also an outdated biology. It may well be that, in the end, we will decide to select boundary markers for protection that are sustained by the best arguments and that are also hallowed by tradition. Or we may choose to shift the lines to take advantage of new research and therapeutic opportunities. But whichever way we go, we will be making a choice. Above all, we must have the honesty and the courage to acknowledge this.

AFTERWORD

A S this book goes to press, a new phase of embryo research is about to begin, and with it, a new set of professional challenges for me. In July of 2000, I was invited by Michael D. West, president and CEO of Advanced Cell Technology (ACT) in Worcester, Mass., to chair an ethics advisory board (EAB) that he wished to establish to provide oversight for the company's new research initiative in therapeutic cloning. In the year ahead, West explained, ACT hoped to begin research that involved taking donated human oocytes, enucleating them, and inserting into them a selected somatic cell nucleus. After a brief period of development, the resulting clonal embryo would then be disaggregated to produce an ES cell line with the genetic qualities of the somatic cell donor. If this research proves successful, it holds the promise that we may someday be able to provide customized, immunologically compatible tissues or even organs for medical treatment. For example, a youngster suffering from juvenile diabetes might be able to receive new insulin-producing cells to replace those damaged by the disease process. This research also raises some of the most controversial issues discussed in this book, including human cloning and the deliberate creation of embryos for research.[377]

After a week of reflection, I agreed to accept West's invitation. I understood the limits of private corporate EAB's like this but concluded that if we did our work well, the kind of oversight we could offer was far better than no

177

oversight at all. As I was accepting West's invitation, other developments were occurring. In Britain, a report by the chief medical officer's expert group recommended a change in regulations that would permit therapeutic cloning for the purpose of developing stem cell lines.[378] This change was strongly ratified by votes in Parliament in December 2000 and January 2001.[379] On 25 August, 2000, the NIH also released its final proposed guidelines for federal funding for ES cell research.[380] Because these guidelines prohibit the creation of embryos for research, they were already outpaced by British and U.S. private sector developments.

It is unclear that either the NIH's initiatives or ACT's will proceed. The Bush Administration is not supportive of this research.[381] It is also possible that the cloning research proposed by companies like ACT may prove so controversial that it will invite new state or national prohibitions. In any case, research activity and the surrounding ethical discussion are both being raised to a new level of intensity. In some respects, the human embryo research debates are just beginning.

NOTES

Introduction

1. Thomson, James A., et al. Similar work using germinal cells from aborted fetuses was also announced by John Gearhart and others at The Johns Hopkins University: Shamblot, Michael J. et al.

2. Marshall, Eliot.

3. Hanson, Michele A., and Daniel A. Dumesic; Wymelenberg, S., for the Institute of Medicine (1990), p. 15.

4. Abma, J. C. et al.; 7.

5. New York State Task Force on Life and the Law, pp. 13–14.

6. "Infertility among Americans," *Newsletter of the Assisted Reproduction Foundation,* vol. 1 (Fall 1998), p. 1 (quoting a U.S. Department of Health and Human Services study at www.mpr.org).

7. Mason, Mary Martin, "Reasonable Activity," "The Baby Shower," and "Beginner's Luck," pp. 13–19, 41–47, 69–76; Liebmann-Smith, Joan, "Infertility 9-to-5," pp. 81–96.

8. Kleiman, Dena.

9. New York State Task Force on Life and the Law, pp. 427–435. For a persuasive defense of insurance for infertility treatments, see Brock, Dan W. (1996).

10. For an influential discussion of what constitutes a disease condition (or what the authors term a "malady"), see Culver, Charles, and Bernard Gert, chapters 4 and 5.

11. The NIH FY 1999 appropriation passed by Congress and signed into law 21 October 1998 (as part of Public Law 105–277) was $15,612,386,000. Of this, the National Institute of Child Health & Human Development, the principal institute funding research on human reproduction, received $752.2 million (audited). Of that $752.2 million, NICHD spent $16.3 million on infertility research. This represents 2.2 percent of its budget and .01 percent of the total NIH budget. Source of NICHD numbers: personal communication with Art Fried of NICHD, 24 February 2000.

12. "Final Report, Survey of Assisted Reproductive Technology: Embryo Laboratory Procedures and Practices," 29 January 1999. Prepared for Centers for Disease Control and Prevention by Analytical Sciences, Inc., Durham, NC. (Website: www.cdc.gov/nccdphp/drh/art.htm).

13. Saunders, K., J. Spensley, J. Munro, G. Halasz; Bernasko, J., L. Lynch, R. Lapinski, and R. L. Berkowitz; "Impact of Multiple Births on Low Birthweight—

Massachusetts, 1989–1996," *MMWR Weekly,* 48/14 (16 April 1999), 289–292; Wilcox, L. S., J. L. Kiely, C. L. Melvin, and M. C. Martin.

14. Centers for Disease Control and Prevention et al., p. 14.

15. Moore, Keith L., and T.V.N. Persaud, p. 34. Also, Carlson, Bruce M. (1994), p. 27.

16. Van Steirteghem, André C.

17. Kolata, Gina (23 December 1999), A1.

18. Wilmut, Ian, Keith Campbell, and Colin Tudge, p. 293.

19. Silver, Lee, p. 8.

Chapter 1

20. Consultants to the Advisory Committee to the Director, National Institutes of Health.

21. 45 Code of Federal Regulations § 46.203.

22. *Newsletter of the Assisted Reproduction Foundation,* vol. 1 (Fall 1998), 1.

23. Mason, Mary Martin, "Reasonable Activity," "The Baby Shower," "Beginner's Luck," pp. 13–19, 41–47, 69–76; Liebmann-Smith, Joan.

24. The actual cost for each accomplished birth is even greater. See Neumann, Peter J. et al.

25. Ethics Advisory Board, Department of Health, Education and Welfare.

26. Mass mailings organized by religious groups have predominated in all recent NIH panel processes dealing with regulations governing embryo or fetal research. The great majority of letters sent to the NIH in connection with the Human Embryo Research Panel reflected Roman Catholic diocesan campaigns. The same appears to be true for public comment on the NIH's recently published proposed human pluripotent stem cell guidelines (personal communication from an official of the NIH Office of Science Policy, 21 February 2000).

27. According to Robert Cook-Deegan, the ethics advisory board was allowed to expire because its function was (mistakenly) believed about to be assumed by the newly created President's Commission for the Study of Ethical Problems in Medicine and Biomedical and Behavioral Research. See Cook-Deegan, p. 259.

28. In July 1988 Robert Windom, assistant secretary for health, announced that a new EAB would be established. A draft of the charter was published in the *Federal Register* for comments, but no further action was taken. The incoming Bush administration never acted on these initiatives. See Norman, C.

29. (NIH) Revitalization Act of 1993 (Pub. L. No 103–43, Sec. 492A. [10 June 1993]). The NIH Revitalization Act nullified the requirement for an ethics advisory board's approval for protocols involving IVF.

30. See Consultants to the Advisory Committee to the Director, National Institutes of Health, "Report of the Human Fetal Tissue Transplantation Research Panel (December 1988)," dissents by Rabbi J. David Bleich, James Bopp, James T. Burtchaell, and Daniel N. Robinson, pp. 39–73.

31. For a discussion of the importance and limits of consensus in the work of public ethics panels, see Benjamin, Martin.

32. Darly A. (Sandy) Chamblee, letter to Senator Bob Graham, 15 April 1994.

33. Tauer, Carol A. (1995), p. 31.

34. 45 CFR § 46.203.

35. A. McClaren in CIBA Foundation, pp. 5–23.

36. National Commission for the Protection of Human Subjects of Biomedical and Behavioral Research, p. 18; Vaheri, A. et al.

37. See introduction, n. 13.

38. Scott, R. T. Jr. et al.

39. Stansberry, J. For a slightly different estimate of the male–female contribution reporting a 40–50 percent female factor, 30–40 percent male factor, and 10–30 percent unexplained or both partners, see http://health.yahoo.com/health/Diseases—and—Conditions/Disease—Feed—Data/Infertility. At this site select "Causes, Incidence, and Risk Factors."

40. Studies of this issue have come to conflicting conclusions. See Bonduelle, M. et al.; Kurinczuk, J. J., and C. Bower.

41. Kolata, Gina (23 December 1999). Online edition: http://www.nytimes.com.

42. Van Steirteghem, André C.

43. Bonaccorsi, A. C. et al.; Wilkins-Haug, L. E., M. S. Rein, and M. D. Hornstein.

44. See note 13.

45. Friedler, S., S. Mashiach, N. Laufer.

46. Human Fertilisation and Embryology Authority. Parts 7–9 stipulate that "no more than three eggs or embryos should be placed in a woman in any one cycle, regardless of the procedure used." For a review of other proposed and existing regulations and standards of practice, see New York State Task Force on Life and the Law, pp. 151–154.

47. Ibid., p. 155.

48. Vatican, Congregation for the Doctrine of the Faith. See also Doerflinger, Richard (1999b), "Testimony Doerflinger, Richard."

49. Corea, Gena; Raymond, J. G., p. 2; Nelson, H. L., 129, 133. For overviews of feminist discussions of ARTs, see Donchin, Anne; and Lebacqz, Karen.

50. Rothman, Barbara Katz, pp. 17–64, 140–151.

51. John Fletcher reports that in September 1979, Patricia Harris, secretary, DHEW, refused to begin the process needed to establish an ethics advisory board for embryo research because she mainly saw IVF as a procedure for the advantaged. See Fletcher, John, p. E-11, note 98.

52. Koch, Lene. Ruth Macklin considers and rejects the overpopulation objection to assisted reproductive technologies in the context of developing countries. See Macklin, Ruth. For a similar presentation and review of these arguments, see Brock, Dan (1996).

53. Culver, Charles, and Bernard Gert, chapters 4 and 5.

54. For a review of this literature, see New York State Task Force on Life and the Law, pp. 117–118, 123.

55. Ibid., p. 117.

56. In July 1998 the federal government ruled that states must provide coverage for Viagra through Medicaid programs, which cover other prescription drugs. See Porter, Rebecca. Some justified this spending on the grounds that a healthy sex life is fundamental to well-being. See Barada, James.

57. See notes 7 and 8.

58. See notes 4 and 5.

59. For a discussion of the difficulties adoption poses for couples facing infertility, see "The Myth and Reality of Current Adoption Practices" in Lauritzen, Paul, pp. 119–134.

60. See note 5.

61. Non-Hispanic white women are twice as likely as white women, and four times as likely as black women, to have used ARTs. See Abma, J. C. et al., 65.

62. The incidence of infertility is 10.5 percent among married couples for non-Hispanic black women, roughly 1.5 times greater than among Hispanic or non-Hispanic white women—ibid., 61; see also Washington, Harriet.

63. 36 U.S. 535 (1942).

64. 381 U.S. 479 (1965).

65. 410 U.S. 113 (1973).

66. *Lifchez* v. *Hartigan* 735 F. Suppl. 1361 (N.D. Ill.), *aff'd*, 914 F.2d 260 (7th Cir. 1990), *cert. denied*, 498 U.S. 1069 (1991). According to the court, "It takes no great leap of logic to see that within the cluster of constitutionally protected choices that includes the right to have access to contraceptives, there must be included within that cluster the right to submit to a medical procedure that may bring about, rather than prevent, pregnancy" (at 1377).

67. Robertson, John (1994).

68. Brock, Dan W. (1996).

69. As early as 1988, a report prepared for Congress by the Office of Technology Assessment (OTA) stated: "The effect of this moratorium on federal funding of IVF research has been to eliminate the most direct line of authority by which the Federal Government can influence the development of embryo research and infertility treatment so as to avoid unacceptable practices or inappropriate uses. It has also dramatically affected the financial ability of American researchers to pursue improvements in IVF and the development of new infertility treatments, possibly affecting in turn the development of new contraceptives based on improved understanding of the process of fertilization." U.S. Congress, Office of Technology Assessment, p. 179. See also Blank, R. H.

70. It is estimated that inherited genetic disorders account for one-quarter to one-third of children admitted to pediatric units in Western nations. See Brent, R. L. See also "Early Diagnosis and Prevention of Genetic Disease," in Galjaard, H., p. 1.

71. Jos, P. H., M. F. Marshall and M. Perlmutter.

72. Crosby, U. D., B. E. Schwartz, K. L. Gluck, S. F. Heartwell; Alfa, Michelle J., Jeffrey J. Sisler, and Godfrey K. M. Harding; Sarma Seshu P., and Robert P. Hatcher. On 26 August 1999 Norplant's manufacturer, American Home Products Corporation, settled a lawsuit by 36,000 women claiming to have been inadequately warned about such side effects. See Morrow, David J.

73. The name of this organization has recently been changed to the National Catholic Bioethics Center.

74. Catholic teaching permits some forms of clinical embryo research so long as they are "used for the benefit of the embryo itself in a final attempt to save its life and in the absence of other forms of reliable therapy." See Vatican, Congregation for the Doctrine of the Faith, p. 703.

75. Doerflinger continues to voice this criticism. See Doerflinger, Richard (1999a), "The Ethics of . . . ," p. 146.

76. Human Embryo Research Panel, meeting transcript, 2 February 1994, p. 94.

77. Ibid., p. 93.

78. A special interdisciplinary commission is currently at work at the Vatican to help the Roman Catholic church form a position on when death may be thought to occur. The imprecision of Catholic teaching on the time of death is reflected in standard encyclopedia discussions. See, for example, Delaney, Joseph F.; and Osburn, R. A.

79. The official teaching of the church on this matter is not much more precise than was Father May. Vatican Congregation for the Doctrine of the Faith, "Donum Vitae" ("Instruction on Respect for Human Life in Its Origin and on the Dignity of Procreation,") states ". . . in the zygote (the cell produced when the nuclei of the two gametes have fused) resulting from fertilization the biological identity of a new human individual is already constituted." See p. 701.

80. Andrews's testimony was derived from two papers prepared for the panel. One, written by Andrews and Nanette Elster, "Cross-Cultural Analysis of Policies Regarding Embryo Research," deals with legislation and policies in other countries. The other, "State Regulation of Embryo Research," focuses on U.S. state laws and the reports of some professional committees. These two papers (with their extensive appendixes of laws and reports) appear respectively as pp. 51–296 and 297–407 in National Institutes of Health, *Papers Commissioned for the Human Embryo Research Panel*. For another summary of the state laws governing human embryo research, see New York State Task Force on Life and the Law, pp. 386–387.

81. Andrews, Lori and Nanette Elster, p. 53.

82. *La. Rev. Stat. Ann.* § 9:122 (West 1997).

83. Steinbock, Bonnie (1994a). Steinbock's position is more fully developed in her earlier book (1992) and a more recent chapter (2001).

84. Locke, John, pp. 211, 220. For a fuller discussion of the various uses of the concept "humanity," see Bok, Sissela.

Chapter 2

85. Green, Ronald M. (1967, 1974, 1983, 1998).

86. Green, Ronald M. (1983).

87. The following description of the fertilization process is drawn from Carlson, Bruce M. (1994), pp. 27–32. The attractive role of the egg is signaled by Carlson and in recent studies by David Garbers of the University of Texas Southwestern Medical School. Garbers reports that small peptide molecules emitted by the egg bind to a receptor protein on the sperm's surface and have a "dramatic, attractive effect" causing it to move toward the egg. See http://www.hhmi.org/science/cellbio/egg.htm/.

88. Carlson, Bruce M. (1994), p. 29.

89. Austin, C. R., p. 9, estimates the rate of polyspermic fertilization at about 2 percent. See also Sadler, T. W., p. 27; Moore, Keith L., and T.V.N. Persaud, p. 37.

90. This is in addition to a first polar body that is already outside the egg cytoplasm and that is produced during the first division of meiosis.

91. Australia (Victoria). The Infertility (Medical Procedures) (Amendment) Act 1987, 9a (1). For a discussion of the legislative and other debates around this issue, see Buckle, Stephen, Karen Dawson, and Peter Singer.

92. O'Rahilly, Ronan, and Fabiola Müller, p. 20: "The two pronuclei do not fuse but their nuclear envelopes break down and form vesicles." For the physical contrast here between the zygote and two cell stage, see Sadler, T. W., p. 29, figures 2–7.

93. Ian Wilmut and Keith Campell stress the fact that cloned embryos, which contain a single, inserted diploid nucleus, differ in this respect from normal zygotes, which never contain a single nucleus but only two separated pronuclei. They observe that this difference of detail may someday be regarded as being of practical importance. See "The Facts of Life Revisited" in Wilmut, Ian, Keith Campbell, and Colin Tudge, p. 105.

94. Ibid., pp. 125, 172.

95. Carlson, Bruce M. (1994), p. 27; see also Moore, Keith L., and T.V.N. Persaud, p. 34; O'Rahilly, Ronan, and Fabiola Müller, p. 19: "Fertilization is the procession of events that begins when a spermatozoan makes contact with a secondary oocyte or its investments, and ends with the intermingling of maternal and paternal chromosomes at metaphase of the first mitotic division of the zygote."

96. Kolata, Gina (1993); Massey, J. B., M. J. Tucker, H. J. Malter, and J. L. Hall.

97. Willadsen, S. M. (1981); Willadsen, S. M. (1989).

98. Huxley, Aldous.

99. Bulmer puts the natural rate of monozygotic twinning at 3.4 per thousand maternities and the natural frequency of monozygotic triplets at about 20 per million. See Bulmer, M. G., pp. 3, 98.

100. O'Rahilly, Ronan, and Fabiola Müller, p. 6.

101. Austin, C. R., p. 17.

102. Harper, J. C., and A. H. Handyside; Müller, Hansjakob.

103. Strain, Lisa ,John C. S. Dean, Mark P. R. Hamilton, and David T. Bonthron.

104. Lockwood, Michael.

105. Ford, Norman M., pp. 102–118; McCormick, R. A; Shannon, Thomas and Allan B. Woltor. Influential earlier statements of this position include Hellegers, André; and Diamond, James.

106. Human Embryo Research Panel, meeting transcript, 2 February 1994, p. 8.

107. Shannon, Thomas and Allan B. Woltor, 620; see also, Bobik, J.

108. Moraczewski, Albert S., pp. 52–53.

109. This view would be supported by the traditional Roman Catholic perspective (drawn from Aristotle) known as hylomorphism, according to which spiritual events require an appropriate material substrate. For centuries before the modern era, such a view underlay Roman Catholic thinking on fetal ensoulment, which was believed to occur in stages. For an account of this position, see Donceel, Joseph. See also Shannon, Thomas and Allan B. Woltor, 614–619.

110. Morison, Robert.

111. Zaner, Richard M, pp. 17–74. For a discussion of those jurisdictions where, for religious reasons, brain death has not been fully accepted, see Veatch, Robert M., chapter 2.

112. I am not considering here whether our philosophical conception or "definition" of death has also been changed by technology. Instead, I am focusing on various criteria for identifying when death has occurred. However, I believe that our basic definition of death is also subject to value-based revision. This is indicated by the fact that various debates over higher or lower brain death depend on competing notions of what makes human life worth living. For a discussion of the distinction between a definition of death and criteria for determining death, see Bernat, James, pp. 113–143.

113. Even Veatch, who recognizes the moral dimension of using the term "irreversible" when applied to other biological functions, applies it uncritically to the cessation of brain function. Ibid., pp. 26–27.

114. Fortes, Meyer, p. 266.

115. "Quickening is a phenomenon of maternal perception rather than a fetal achievement." André Hellegers quoted in Noonan, John T., p. 73.

116. This is one reason why there has been continuing discussion of the choice of death as whole-brain, or neocortical, death. See, for example, the President's Commission for the Study of Ethical Problems in Medicine and Biomedical and Behavioral

Research. For an overview of recent discussions about the medical definition and determination of death, see Youngner, S. J., R. M. Arnold, and R. Schapiro.

117. Partly influenced by Orthodox Jewish groups, the state of New Jersey permits some individuals to adopt a cardiac definition of death for themselves or loved ones. See Veatch, Robert M., p. 27. In Japan, Buddhist and Shinto beliefs contributed to this reluctance to accept brain death. Only in early 1997 did Japanese law permit recovering hearts and other organs for transplant from brain dead patients kept alive on respirators. See "The Law Concerning Organ Transplants (The Law of No. 104 in 1997)" at http://www.kuleuven.ac.be/facdep/medicine/icts/latest/japan.html.

118. An estimate for early embryo loss of between 69 percent and 78 percent is given by Biggers, J. D., in his testimony, p. 11. Roberts, C. J., and C. R. Lowe offer a "conservative estimate" that in England and Wales married women aged 20–29 may abort 78 percent of their conceptions. A much lower rate of 33 percent is offered by Larsen, William J., p. 22. O'Rahilly, Ronan, and Fabiola Müller, p. 56, state that up to 40 percent of embryos under four weeks of age do not go on to develop. However, they estimate the total loss of conceptuses from fertilization to birth at between 50 percent and 80 percent.

119. Larsen, William J., p. 22. O'Rahilly, Ronan, and Fabiola Müller, p. 56, report that a high percentage of all spontaneously aborted conceptuses (30 percent to 80 percent, depending on the study) are structurally abnormal, while all abortuses under four postovulatory weeks have abnormally formed embryonic tissue.

120. Fleck, Leonard M., points out the implications of this high rate of fetal mortality and morbidity for conservative abortion policy.

121. Warren, Mary Anne (1997), p. 3.

122. Dolan, Edwin G.

123. Warren, Mary Anne (1997) discusses many possible criteria for justifying judgments of moral status, but she only fleetingly touches on the fundamental nature of the decision process that leads to these criteria. Well into her discussion (p. 121) she observes that "[m]oral agents 'invent' moral status by reasonably agreeing to accept specific moral obligations to one another—and often toward other beings and things." However, she never systematically lays out the types of considerations that would lead moral agents to accept such obligations as limits on their behavior. Although her multiple criteria of status are an advance over "uni-criterial" approaches, Warren follows most proponents of uni-criterial views in placing emphasis on the results of the status-determining decision process (her multiple criteria and their relation to classes of entities), rather than on the nature of the process that leads to the criteria in the first place. For a more self-reflective, process-oriented approach, see Green, Ronald M. (1983).

124. A similar point is made by Williams, Bernard, pp. 133–134.

125. Buckle, Stephen; Singer, Peter, and Karen Dawson; Warren, Mary Anne (1977) and (1997), pp. 205–208; Watt, Helen; Stone, Jim; and Bigelow, John, and Robert Pargetter.

126. Thompson, Judith J.

127. Victoria, Australia. The Infertility (Medical Procedures) (Amendment) Act 1987, 9a (1).

128. "Je crois bien que, dans tous les domaines de la médicine, celui des techniques d'assistance médicale à la procréation est vraiment le seul où l'on s'autorise aujourd'hui ces expériences dont la réussite ou l'insuccès doivent être directement établis d'après non seulement la survenue d'une grossesse, mais aussi l'état de l'enfant né." See Kahn, Axel.

129. Williams, Bernard.

130. Carlson, Bruce M. (1988), p. 134.

131. Ibid., pp. 457–458. Following a review of the literature on fetal brain development and activity, Burgess, J. A., and S. A. Tawia locate the beginning of consciousness at about 30–35 weeks after conception.

132. Virtually all major moral theories from Kant to Rawls stress that in making moral decisions we must (impartially) consider the impact of our decisions on all other moral agents. It is unclear whether the universality of perspective required by these theories also embraces nonrational human beings and animals. In utilitarianism, the stress on maximizing pleasure and happiness (or minimizing pain and unhappiness) seems to counsel the inclusion of other sentient beings in any calculus of the impacts of our choices. See Sidgwick, Henry, p. 414, and Singer, Peter (1979), p. 19.

133. Englert, Yvon. Englert reports, however, that couples who identified themselves as Roman Catholic were less willing to donate spare embryos to research.

134. A similar conclusion is arrived at by Hare, R. M.

135. Marquis, Don. "Why Abortion is Immoral."

136. For a similar analysis of why we object to killing, see the discussion of the various uses of the concept "humanity" in Bok, Sissela.

137. Marquis, Don, rightly observes that we believe it wrong to kill persons who have little desire to live, no desire to live, or who desire not to live. This includes the unconscious, the sleeping, those who are tired of life, and those who are suicidal. He concludes from this that future life has value regardless of whether it is desired. But each of us could be an unconscious, sleeping, or impulsively suicidal person, and it is only reasonable not to want our lives to be taken against our will or to permit others to kill us in such circumstances. There is no evidence or reason to believe that there exists a similar reasonable desire to preserve the life or prevent the death of early conceptuses.

138. Green, Ronald M., Bernard Gert, and K. Danner Clouser.

139. This perspective may be less prevalent in Asian countries, where Hindu and Buddhist ideas concerning the developmental nature of life prevail. See, for example, Lafleur, William R. See also the special section, "Articles, Review Essay, and Response on the Theme of Mizuko Kuyō in Japan," *Journal of the American Academy of Religion* 67/4 (December 1999), 767–823. This includes articles by LaFleur, Meredith Underwood, Elizabeth Harrison, and Ronald M. Green.

140. Moraczewski, Albert S.

141. Kuhse, Helga, and Peter Singer.

142. Lockwood, Michael (1985); Brody, Baruch; Kovács, Jósef; Veatch, Robert M., pp. 30–32.

143. "[I]t is a necessary condition of something's having a serious right to life that it possesses a concept of a self as a subject of experiences, and that it believes that it is itself such an entity." Tooley, Michael, 47.

144. Singer, Peter (1975 and 1979).

145. Tooley, Michael.

146. Warren, Mary Anne (1973).

147. Similar points are made by Warren, Mary Anne (1997), p. 218.

148. Ibid., pp. 164–165.

149. Singer, Peter (1975).

150. Ibid., p. 75.

151. Childress, James F.; Doerflinger, Richard (1999a), 140.

152. Warnock, Mary. Hare, R. M., p. 188, issues a stinging rebuke of the philosophical argumentation offered by the Warnock committee report, stating that the committee "almost completely shirked the task of offering reasons for its conclusions."

153. Royal Commission on New Reproductive Technologies.

154. Brock, Dan W. (1995b), p. 217.

Chapter 3

155. Smitz, J., et al.

156. The findings to date on the cancer risks of the ovulation-inducing medications widely used in infertility treatments have been unclear or contradictory. One study found that the prolonged use (more than one year) of clomiphene citrate, one of the leading stimulatory medications, more that doubled the expected incidence of borderline or invasive ovarian cancers in a cohort of nearly 4,000 women. Rossing, Mary Anne, et al. Other studies have supported these claims of risk. See, for example, Fuller, Paul N. However, some studies and reviews of studies have questioned whether other, infertility-related problems may not be the cause of these findings: Bristow, Robert E., and Beth Y. Karlan; Paulson, Richard J.

157. Hogan, Brigid; Matsui, Y. et al.; Labosky, P. A., D. P. Barlow, and B. L. Hogan.

158. Human Embryo Research Panel, transcript of meeting, 14 March 1994, p. 25.

159. Ibid., p. 97.

160. Rawls, John (1971), pp. 48–51.

161. The mechanism of contraceptive action of the IUD is still not definitively understood. Some have adduced evidence that the device works by inhibiting fertilization through spermicidal action. See, for example, Oritz, M. E., and H. Croxatto; and Sivin, I. However, a recent review of studies concludes that "the analysis of evidence strongly suggests that the contraceptive effectiveness of intrauterine contraceptive devices is achieved both by a prefertilization spermicidal action and a postfertilization inhibition of uterine implantation." Spinnato, Joseph A.

162. Human Embryo Research Panel, transcript of meeting, 14 March 1994, p. 120.

163. Ibid., p. 121.

164. Ibid.

165. In chapter six of Warren, Mary Anne (1997), she puts forth what she calls a "multi-criterial" approach to the determination of moral status. This is somewhat similar to the pluralistic view I developed in the Human Embryo Research Panel Report and in my earlier writings on abortion, especially my essay "Conferred Rights and the Fetus." Warren and I share the idea that there are a variety of intersecting considerations, not all of which represent intrinsic properties in an entity, that may be invoked in order to justify judgments of moral status. However, Warren's criteria are more like independent moral principles, whereas the plurality of considerations to which I allude describe the basic features of an entity that recommend protecting it given the interests of impartial rational agents. I believe my approach provides the more basic reasoning underlying Warren's criteria.

166. Callahan, Daniel.

167. Englert, Yvon.

168. Callahan, Daniel.

169. Human Embryo Research Panel, transcript of meeting, 14 March 1994, p. 123.

170. One of the recommendations of the New York State Task Force on Life and the Law, p. 174, is that "[n]ew assisted reproductive procedures of unproven safety and efficacy should generally be introduced through a formal research protocol, with the review and approval of an IRB."

Chapter 4

171. Ethics Advisory Board, Department of Health, Education and Welfare, pp. 106–107.

172. Human Fertilisation and Embryology Authority, §§ 5:13, 10:2.

173. Royal Commission on New Reproductive Technologies, vol. 1, pp. 638–641.

174. Council of Europe, article 18.2. See also, Sheldon, Tony.

175. Rossing, Mary Anne et al.; Fuller, Paul N.; Bristow, Robert E. and Beth Y. Karlan; Paulson, Richard J.

176. Stillman, R. J.; Herbst, A. L. et al.; Shy, K. K. et al.

177. Martin, Gwen; "Selling My Eggs," *Glamour Magazine,* May 1994, p. 168; Horovitz, Bruce; Nelkin, Dorothy, and Lori Andrews.

178. Eppig's research in this area is ongoing. For a recent press report, see Travis, John.

179. Edwards, Robert, and Patrick Steptoe, pp. 92–94.

180. Chapter one, p. 10.

181. French, Howard W.

182. Hardacre, Helen, p. 68.

183. Kolata, Gina (1997b).

184. "Women Fight for Right to Fertilise their Frozen Eggs," *The Daily Telegraph,* 16 December 1999; "Baby Hope Dashed for Cancer Victim," *The Guardian,* 16 December 1999: "Woman Starts Legal Battle over Her Eggs," *The Times,* 16 December 1999; "Women at the Mercy of the Foetal Police," *The Guardian,* 17 December 1999.

185. For a discussion of the clinical and ethical issues raised by pregnancies in older women, including postmenopausal women, see New York State Task Force on Life and the Law, pp. 196–200.

186. In 1995 the Genetics and IVF Institute (GIVF) of Fairfax, Virginia, began offering "ovary cryopreservation" for women anticipating radiation or chemotherapy treatments for cancer that would render them sterile. Two years later it expanded its promotion of this service to include women who wished "to protect future child-bearing options that could be limited by ovarian and egg aging." This procedure, which involves the preparation and freezing of thin slices of egg-bearing ovarian tissue, has been successful in sheep, but reimplantation has not yet been attempted in human beings. This commercial offer raises questions concerning the appropriateness of introducing untested procedures into the clinical context. For a discussion of GIVF claims and the controversy around them, see New York State Task Force on Life and the Law, pp. 164–165.

187. No one is sure of the exact number of frozen embryos worldwide. A 1996 estimate by Michael Tucker, scientific director at Reproductive Biology Associates in Atlanta, estimated the number at close to a million. See Maranto, Gina, for Tucker's method of calculation.

188. Tauer, Carol (1997), p. 179.

189. Richard Doerflinger applies the same criticism to reject the use of either spare or research embryos. "If those who object to experiments on embryos created for research would examine more closely the reasons for their moral revulsion, they would find the roots of an argument against destroying embryos regardless of their origins." See Doerflinger, Richard (1999a), pp. 143–145.

190. Kant, Immanuel, p. 46. For an analysis of Kant's position see Green, Ronald (2001).

191. Annas, George, Arthur Caplan, and Sherman Elias, "The Politics of Human-Embryo Research—Avoiding Ethical Gridlock." For a similar view see Ryan, Maura A.

192. Ibid., p. 1331.

193. Draft Report on Human Stem Cell Research, 6 May 1999, p. 18. Quoted by permission of the National Bioethics Advisory Commission.

194. National Bioethics Advisory Commission (1999), vol. 1, pp. 55–56.

195. Human Embryo Research Panel, transcript of meeting, 11 April 1994, p. 87.

196. Ibid., p. 98.

197. Ibid., p. 177.

198. On the $150,000 that some models are charging for their eggs, see Bruce Horovitz, "Selling Beautiful Babies," *USA Today*, 25 October 1999, p. 1A, and Carey Goldberg, "Web Site Selling Models' Eggs," *The Gazette (Montreal)*, 23 October 1999, p. D19. An infertile couple reportedly offered $50,000 for an egg from a tall, athletic college student with high SAT scores, advertising in the student newspapers of top U.S. universities. See "Issues for the 21st Century: The Frontier Within Us," *Boston Globe*, 2 January 2000, p. C6.

199. Human Embryo Research Panel, transcript of meeting, 11 April 1994, pp. 95f.

200. Ibid., p. 87.

201. Ibid., p. 97.

202. Ibid., p. 87.

203. National Institutes of Health (1994a), Appendix A: Statement of Patricia A. King Concurring in Part and Dissenting in Part, pp. A3–A4.

204. 45 Code of Federal Regulations §46.406.

Chapter 5

205. *Junior Lewis Davis* v. *Mary Sue Davis*, no. 34, Supreme Court of Tennessee at Knoxville, 842 S.W.2d 588; 1992 Tenn. 1 June 1992, filed. This case involved a dispute between a divorced husband and wife over the disposition of frozen embryos they had created together in an infertility procedure. LeJeune's testimony aimed at supporting Ms. Davis's wish to gain "custody" over the embryos in order to use them, against her husband's wishes, to continue to try to have a child.

206. Lejeune, Jerome, pp. 28–41.

207. National Institutes of Health (1994a), p. x.

208. Ibid.

209. Quoted in Pence, Gregory E., p. 154. Charo's position here was based on careful study of the European, and specifically the French, alternative. See Charo, Alta, pp. 477–500.

210. We did permit defraying actual expenses incurred by the donor. National Institutes of Health (1994a), p. xi.

211. "Minimum Procurement Standards for an Organ Procurement Organization (OPO), 2.4. Available at www.unos.org.

212. National Institutes of Health (1994a), p. xv.

213. "National Institutes of Health Guidelines for Research Using Human Pluripotent Stem Cells."

214. The issue subsequently became a matter of bioethics debate. See Rubenstein, D. S., D. C. Thomasma, E. A. Schon, and M. J. Zinaman, and Szebik, Imre.

215. The others were Pat King's dissent from our second condition permitting research embryos and Bernie Lo's objection to our permission to use existing embryos for which one of the progenitors was an anonymous gamete donor who had received monetary compensation. We banned the use of such embryos from the time when our report would be accepted by the Advisory Committee to the Director, but made an exception for the many such spare embryos already in existence that would otherwise be wasted. Lo believed that this exception weakened the force of our intended ban. National Institutes of Health (1994a), C-3.

216. Massey, J. B. et al.

217. In January 2000 a team of researchers at the Oregon Primate Center announced the birth of the first primate, a monkey named Tetra, as a result of the embryo splitting technique. Their hope was to produce eventually a genetically uniform line of animals for biomedical research. However, their low success rate—one successful birth in 13 transfers, lower than comparable IVF rates with undivided embryos—provided no reason to believe this would be a useful technology for infertility medicine. See Chan, A. W. S. et al.

218. Marshall, Eliot, "Rules on Human Embryo Research Due Out."

219. "Statement by the President," The White House, Office of the Press Secretary, 2 December 1994.

220. For a related criticism of Clinton's conduct in this matter, see Carmen, Ira H., p. 103. Carmen is particularly critical of Clinton's "cavalier attitude" in abruptly terminating the administration's internal reviews and revisions of the panel's report.

221. See above, chapter 2.

222. The fetal tissue panel's report was approved unanimously by the Advisory Council to the Director of the NIH and submitted to Louis Sullivan, secretary of the Department of Health and Human Services. Nevertheless, its recommendations were rejected by Sullivan in a letter to the panel's chair without any public hearings or prior notification published in the *Federal Register*. For a discussion of this episode, see Fletcher, John C., pp. 45–46.

223. For reviews of the experiences of earlier bioethics commissions, see Gray, Bradford H.

224. Healy took office in April 1991. The Fetal Tissue Transplantation Research Panel issued its report more than two years earlier, in December 1988. This was not acted on either by Healy or her predecessor, James B. Wyngaarden.

225. Public Law 104–99, Section 128, 26 January 1996, 110 Stat 34.

226. Katz, Jeffrey L.

227. Ibid.

Chapter 6

228. See, for example, Green, Ronald M. (1976b); Green, Ronald M. (1976a); Green, Ronald M. (1994a).

229. For more information on the Human Genome Project and the role of the NIH and other government agencies, visit the project's web site: http://www.ornl.gov/ TechResources/Human_Genome/home.html. It was originally planned that the full human genome would be sequenced by the year 2003. However, in December 1999, Craig Venter, head of Celera Genomics, announced that his company would be in a position to publish the full sequence later in 2000. On 26 June 2000 the "final assembly" of the genome was announced in a White House ceremony presided over by President Clinton. Francis Collins spoke for the public program and Venter represented Celera. For an account of the infighting that preceded this resolution, see Preston, Richard.

230. For a discussion of this problem, see Rothenberg, Karen H.

231. Public Law 104-99, section 128, January 26 1996, 110 Stat 34. Currently, the ban appears as section 511 of the "Omnibus Consolidated and Emergency Supplemental Appropriations, Fiscal Year 1999," Public Law 105–277, October 1998.

232. 45 Code of Federal Regulations §46.208(a)(2).

233. 45 Code of Federal Regulations §46.406.

234. Along with its ban on funding for embryo research, Congress also reaffirmed its prohibition on federal funding (with three exceptions) for elective abortions in the Medicaid program. Public Law 104–34, section 131, 26 April 1996, 110 Stat 1321–82.

235. Wilmut, I., et al.

236. Wilmut, I.

237. For an account of the research leading to the birth of Dolly, see Wilmut, Ian, Keith Campbell, and Colin Tudge.

238. Cole-Turner, Ronald. The Roman Catholic church, the Southern Baptist Convention, and the United Methodist church called for a ban of human cloning. Jewish leaders, on the other hand, have been reluctant to do so, claiming the arguments that might be marshaled against cloning are not adequately convincing. Other Protestant groups have refrained from making a judgment. See Gayle White, "Is Cloning Mastermind Playing God?," *Atlanta Constitution*, 11 January 1998, p. 1A. See also, Sylvia Brooks, "Cloning Raises Host of Issues for Theologians," *Columbus Dispatch*, 25 February 1997, p. 1A; Kari Leif Bates and Tom Greenwood, "Sheep Now; Humans Next?: Cloning Breakthrough Fuels Ethical, Religious Debate," *Detroit News*, 25 February 1997, p. A1; Ken Symon, "Churchmen Call for Treaty on Cloning," *Sunday Times*, 11 May 1997; Cecile S. Holmes, "Southern Baptists Propose Bans on Human Cloning," *Houston Chronicle*, 20 June 1997, p. 4; Graeme Stewart, "Catholic Church Questions Ethics of Roslin Cloning Work," *The Scotsman*, 29 April 1998, p. 8; Gerald L. Zelizer, "Religious Leaders Rush Too Quickly to Ban Cloning," *USA Today*, 27 July 1998, p. 1; Ronald A. Lindsay, "Taboos Without a Clue," *Free Inquiry*, 17/3 (Summer 1997), 15–17.

239. In January 1998 nineteen nations signed a treaty, which was drafted by the United States, Japan, Canada, and the Vatican, to ban human cloning. The countries that signed were Denmark, Estonia, Finland, France, Greece, Iceland, Italy, Latvia, Luxembourg, Macedonia, Moldova, Norway, Portugal, Romania, San Marino, Slovenia, Spain, Sweden, and Turkey: "19 Nations Sign Treaty to Ban Cloning of Humans," *Buffalo News*, 13 January 1998, p. 1A; M. Wadman, "Cloning for Research Should Be Allowed," *Nature* 388 (1997), 6; Reuters, "WHO Says Cloning Would Be Unethical." at http://www.yahoo.com/headlines, 11 March 1997.

240. Seelye, K. Q.

241. A few of those who introduced such bills include Rep. Vernon J. Ehlers (R.-Mich.) for 1997 HR 923, Sen. Ben Nighthorse Campbell (R.-Colo.) for 1998 5 1574,

Sen. Trent Lott (R.-Miss.) for 1998 5 1601, State Senator John Marchi (R.-Staten Island), and Sen. Dianne Feinstein (D.-Calif.) for 1998 5 1602. See Dan Carney, "Most Adopting Cautious Approach as Congress Confronts Cloning," *CQ Weekly* (on-line), 15 March 1997; Vernon J. Ehlers, "Ban Human Cloning," *USA Today*, 18 June 1997, p. 14A; Jeff Nesmith, "Focus on Human Cloning," *Atlanta Constitution*, 8 January 1998, p. 3E; and "State Senator Proposes Legislation to Ban Cloning Humans," *Buffalo News*, 12 January 1998, p. 4A.

242. See Rick Weiss, "Scientist Plans to Clone Humans," *Washington Post*, 7 January 1998, p. A3; Steve Sternberg, "Human Cloning Seed Sees a World with Disease-Free Children," *USA Today*, 8 January 1998, p. 1A; Richard Saltus, "Would-Be Cloner Plans to Start with Himself," *Boston Globe*, 6 September 1998, p. A6; and Sharon Kirkey, "Richard Seed: The Face of Human Cloning," *The Ottawa Citizen*, 15 October 1999, p. A1.

243. National Bioethics Advisory Commission (1997).

244. For negative evaluations of cloning in terms of the impact on the child, see ibid., chapters 3 and 4, especially the positions mentioned there that have been articulated by Haas, Meilaender, Verhey, the Pope John Center, and Jonas.

245. This position was voiced before the commission by Lisa Cahill and challenged by Protestant theologian Nancy Duff. Ibid., pp. 53–54.

246. Ibid., p. 57.

247. Ibid., pp. 57, 74–75.

248. Wilmut, Ian, Keith Campbell, and Colin Tudge, p. 216.

249. National Bioethics Advisory Commission (1997), p. 24; Kolata, Gina, (1998), pp. 239–242; Wilmut, Ian, Keith Campbell, and Colin Tudge, p. 293. A very recent report, however, suggests that cloning actually increases the length of telomeres in bovines. This suggests that the shortened telomeres seen in Dolly may be species-specific. See Lanza, R. P. et al. (2000a).

250. National Bioethics Advisory Commission (1997), p. ii.

251. Ibid., p. 109.

252. Bonnicksen, Andrea L., 25.

253. This point is made by Kahn, Jeffrey P., 33.

254. Religious ethicists and theologians formed the majority of the twelve invited speakers. They included Lisa Cahill (Roman Catholicism), Elliot Dorff (Judaism), Nancy Duff (Protestantism), Gilbert C. Meilaender, Jr. (Protestantism), Albert S. Moraczewski (Roman Catholicism), Abdulaziz Sachedina (Islam), and Moshe Tendler (Judaism).

255. Campbell, Courtney S. (1997).

256. National Bioethics Advisory Commission (1997), pp. 39–40. The report here itemizes the reasons why religious thinkers were invited to play a role in the deliberation process.

257. This point is made by Campbell, Courtney (1999), in his defense of NBAC's appeal to religious perspectives, 34.

258. Charo, Alta (1997), 16. Also, her remarks quoted in Kolata, Gina (1997a), p. C9. In a previously published discussion, Charo had voiced her criticism of the approach to moral reasoning taken by the Human Embryo Research Panel. See Charo, Alta (1995b).

259. Lewontin, Richard.

260. Green, Ronald (1987).

261. Five of the six statements issued by denominational bodies that are reprinted

in Siker, Jeffrey S., pp. 195–208, take a negative view of homosexuality and deny ordination to non-celibate homosexual persons.

262. National Bioethics Advisory Commission (1997), p. 57.

263. Positive views on cloning were principally voiced by Jewish and Islamic spokespeople. For a discussion of why Jewish thinkers are more positive about the new reproductive technologies, see Green, Ronald M. (1999a) and (1999b).

264. Robertson, John A. (1998).

265. In House hearings on proposed cloning legislation, Alison Taunton-Rigby noted that one of the prohibitory bills being proposed required confiscation of "any property . . . used to commit a violation." She asked whether this bill would permit confiscation of an entire university, certainly a chilling consideration for any research bordering on cloning. See Taunton-Rigby, Alison, p. 82.

266. See Charo, Alta (1997), 16–17.

267. Letter from Harold T. Shapiro, (chair of the National Bioethics Advisory Commission) to the president of 9 June 1997. This appears with the prefatory material in National Bioethics Advisory Commission (1997).

268. National Bioethics Advisory Commission (1997), p. 65.

269. Examples include 1997: 105 H.R.922, 105 H.R. 923; 1998: 105 H.R. 3133, 105 S. 1574, 105 S. 1601, 105 S. 1602; 1999: 106 H.R. 2326, and 106 H.R. 571.

270. Kass, Leon R.

271. A similar position is developed in Heyd, David. Other treatments of this issue, some coming to different conclusions from Parfit and Heyd, include Feinberg, Joel (1992); Woodward, J.; Bigelow, John, and Robert Pargetter; Hanser, M.; Harris, John (1992), chapter 4; Brock, D. W. (1995a) and (2000); Heller, J. C.; ed., and Fotion, Nick and Jan C. Heller.

272. Parfit, Derek, part 4. For a roughly similar approach, see Brock, D. W. (1995a) and (2000), pp. 204–257.

273. Bigelow, John, and Robert Pargetter; Singer, Peter (1979), pp. 106–126, and (1976).

274. Narveson, Jan.

275. *Curlender* v. *Bio-Science Laboratories,* Court of Appeal of California, Second Appellate District, Division One, 106 Cal. App. 3d 811; 1980 Cal. App. LEXIS 1919; 165 Cal. Rptr. 477, 11 June 1980.

276. Jecker, N. S.; Peters, P. G., Jr.; Kelly, M. B.; Jackson, Anthony.

277. *Gleitman* v. *Cosgrove,* Supreme Court of New Jersey, 49 N.J. 22; 227 A.2d 689; 1967 N.J. LEXIS 203; 22 A.L.R.3d 1411, 6 March 1967. (Weintraub C. J., dissenting in part) at 72.

278. *Becker* v. *Schwartz et al.,* Court of Appeals of New York, 46 N.Y.2d 401 at 411; 386 N.E.2d 807; 1978 N.Y. LEXIS 2463; 413 N.Y.S.2d 895, 27 December 1978.

279. *Curlender* v. *Bio-Science Laboratories; Turpin,* v. *Sortini et al.,* Supreme Court of California, 31 Cal. 3d 220; 643 P.2d 954; 1982 Cal. LEXIS 170; 182 Cal. Rptr. 337, 3 May 1982; *Harbeson et al.,* v. *Parke-Davis,* Supreme Court of Washington, 98 Wash. 2d 460; 656 P.2d 483; 1983 Wash. LEXIS 1334, 6 January 1983; *Procanik et al.,* v. *Cillo et al.,* Supreme Court of New Jersey, 113 N.J. 357; 550 A.2d 466; 1988 N.J. LEXIS 1013, 27 September 1988. In *Curlender* the court rejected "the notion that a 'wrongful life' cause of action involves any attempted evaluation of a claimed right *not* to be born" (at 830–831). It awarded damages to the infant, but only for the pain and suffering in its shortened life, not for the full, normal lifespan its parents claimed it had been denied. In *Turpin* the court permitted recovery for the extraordinary, addi-

tional medical expenses involved in raising the child. In *Harbeson* the court rejected recovery for general damages but permitted the child to recover the extraordinary expenses to be incurred during the its lifetime. In *Procanik* the court permitted the infant to recover as special damages the extraordinary medical expenses attributable to his affliction but not general damages for emotional distress or for an impaired childhood.

280. *Zeitzov* v. *Katz* (1986) 40(ii) P.D. 45. This case is discussed by David Heyd in his *Genethics*, p. 27. In a recent case a French court awarded damages to a handicapped teenager for "having been born."—"Damages for 'Life Not Worth Living'" *The Times* (London), 18 November 2000, p. 1.

281. Robertson, John A. (1994), p. 117; (1997); and (1998). For a similar defense of cloning as not being harmful to a child who would not otherwise have been born, see Orentlicher, David.

282. Robertson, John A. (1998).

283. J. A. Robertson, "A Ban on Cloning and Cloning Research is Unjustified," testimony presented to the National Bioethics Advisory Commission, 14 March 1997. Quoted in National Bioethics Advisory Commission (1997), p. 66.

284. Ibid.

285. Robertson, John A. (1997).

286. Brock, Dan W. (1995b), p. 234.

287. A number of philosophical discussions of this issue have been published that NBAC might have referenced to buttress its rejection of the argument that it is morally permissible to inflict pain and suffering on a child, provided that the alternative is never to have been conceived (see National Bioethics Advisory Commission (1997), p. 65). These include Purdy, L. M.; Steinbock, Bonnie, and R. McClamrock; Cohen, Cynthia B.

288. Cohen, Cynthia B., 21. I agree with Cohen's conclusions against those arrived at by Roberts, Melinda. Roberts argues that our "well-being in a world in which we exist is higher (at least, likely to be higher) than it is in a world in which we do not exist" (p. 73).

289. Roberts, Melinda, p. 234, argues that such minor genetic differences are inconsequential. However, against this claim, it can be said that even small genetic changes, such as fertilization by an x- rather than a y-bearing sperm, can fundamentally alter the child's life experience.

290. *Wisconsin* v. *Yoder* 406 U.S. 205, 207 (1972).

291. *U.A.W.* v. *Johnson Controls, Inc.* 499 U.S. 187 (1991).

292. This view is challenged by those who believe that parents have strict obligations not to compromise the future autonomy of their child. See, for example, Feinberg, Joel, (1980) and Davis, Dena S.

293. For fuller accounts of this idea, see Green, Ronald M. (1998), chapter 1, and (1994b), chapters 2 and 3. See also Green, Ronald M., Bernard Gert, and K. Danner Clouser.

Chapter 7

294. Thomson, James A. et al., and Shamblot, Michael J. et al.

295. Carol Tauer wrote one of the report's few dissents, arguing for a total ban on the use of research embryos for this purpose. Carol objected to this because she

believed that "[w]hile there may be therapeutic reasons for developing cell lines of a vast variety of genotypes, stem cell research studies do not require that cells be utilized from such a variety of genotypes." Providing this variety of tissue in the future, she maintained, is a task for tissue banks and distribution networks, not one that requires federal support. National Institutes of Health (1994a), Appendix B, "Statement of Carol A. Tauer." The debate about whether the federal government should fund studies on the creation of autologous stem cell lines from research embryos has been accentuated by recent stem cell discoveries.

296. Pollack, Andrew (explaining how Geron Corp. started and developed as a medical research company).

297. The University of Wisconsin Bioethics Advisory Committee also issued a statement approving Thomson's research.

298. "A Statement on Human Embryonic Stem Cells by the Geron Advisory Board," signed by Karen Lebacqz, EAB chair, Michael Mendiola, Ted Peters, Ernlé Young, and Laurie Zoloth-Dorfman. A later version of this statement appears as "Research with Human Embryonic Stem Cells: Ethical Considerations," *Hastings Center Report* 29/2 (1999), 31–36

299. A series of discussions of the Geron board appears as "Symposium: Human Primordial Stem Cells," *Hastings Center Report* 29/2 (1999), 30–48. At a recent pubic forum on stem cell research at the annual meeting of the American Academy for the Advancement of Science (21 February 2000), John Gearhart explained why he resorted to Geron's funding, even though NIH funding of EG cell research was legally possible. "Every time I called the program office at NIH," he said, "they weren't there." This experience perhaps reflects the reluctance of NIH administrators to become involved in the funding of EG or ES cell research in the current uncertain legal climate.

300. White, Gladys B.

301. Tauer, Carol A. (1999).

302. Early in 2000 Geron received a U.K. patent on Roslin's cloning technology and filed for a related patent in the United States. See Vogel, Gretchen (2000).

303. Lecture given at the American Academy for the Advancement of Science in Washington, D.C., 25 August 1999, at a public forum sponsored by the AAAS and Institute for Civil Society, "Stem Cell Research & Applications: Scientific, Ethical, and Policy Issues."

304. Vogel, Gretchen (1999); Floyd E. Bloom, "Editorial: Breakthroughs 1999," *Science* 286 (17 December 1999), 2267. Harold Varmus offered a good overview of the possible uses of stem cell research in his testimony before a Senate subcommittee. This was issued by the NIH as "Statement of Harold Varmus, M.D. Director, National Institutes of Health. Before the Senate Appropriations Subcommittee on Labor, Health and Human Services, Education and Related Agencies, January 26, 1999."

305. Specifically, their inherited genetic imprinting, the gene-controlling factors conferred differently by the male and female gametes, has been erased to prepare them for their role in reproduction, when new imprinting takes place. This absence of imprinting appears to lead to abnormal development in mouse embryos into which EG cells have been inserted. See Steghaus-Kovac, Sabine.

306. 45 CF § 46.210.

307. Marshall, Eliot.

308. Letter to Harold Shapiro, 14 November 1998. The president was also concerned about reports that researchers associated with Advanced Cell Technology in

Worcester, Mass. had attempt to fuse a human cell with a cow egg. Wade, Nicholas (1998).

309. Hall, Stephen S.; see also Lanza, Robert P., Jose P. Cibelli, and Michael D. West.

310. Michael West maintains that all bovine genetic material, including that associated with the cow egg mitochondria, is replaced by human material in the resulting embryo in a matter of weeks (personal communication, 29 January 2000). The possibility remains that residual bovine proteins will influence the development of the human DNA and RNA.

311. Nagy, Andràs et al.

312. Kolata, Gina (1999a).

313. Memorandum from Harriet S. Rabb to Harold Varmus. "Federal Funding for Research Involving Human Pluripotent Stem Cells," 15 January 1999.

314. Fiscal Year 1999, Public Law 105–255, Section 511.

315. 5th ed., 1994, p. 1408.

316. John Fletcher, in a paper written to assist NBAC in its deliberations, states that the Rabb memorandum "loudly begs the question of the morality of derivation." "Deliberating Incrementally on Human Pluripotential Stem Cell Research," p. E-5.

317. Letter to the Honorable Donna E. Shalala dated 11 February 1999 and signed by Congressman Jay Dickey et al.

318. Private communication from Michael West of Advanced Cell technology.

319. For a review of the background of this controversy, see Charatan, Fred B.

320. Seidelman, William E. (1989) and (1996); Post, Stephen G.; Caplan, Arthur L.; Moe, Kristine; Velvl W. Greene, "Can Scientists Use Information Derived from the Concentration Camps? Ancient Answers to New Questions," and Nancy L. Segal, "Twin Research at Auschwitz-Birkenau: Implications for the Use of Nazi Data Today," both in Caplan, Arthur L. (1992), pp. 155–170 and 281–299.

321. For a critique of such use of the Holocaust analogy in the context of the abortion debate, see the reply to James Bopp, Jr.'s, dissent by Dr. Aron A. Moscona in Consultants to the Advisory Committee to the Director, National Institutes of Health, *Report of the Human Fetal Tissue Transplantation Research Panel,* December 1988, pp. 27–28. Bopp offers a response to Moscona in Bopp, James, Jr., p. 65.

322. Consultants to the Advisory Committee to the Director, National Institutes of Health, *Report of the Human Fetal Tissue Transplantation Research Panel,* December 1988, p. 3.

323. See Phillips, P.; Kordower, J. H. et al.; Freed, C. R., B. R. Breeze, and S. A. Schenck; Olanow, C. W., J. H. Kordower, T. B. Freeman.

324. Ibrahim, Youssef M.

325. James Bopp, Jr., uses this agent analogy in his criticism of fetal tissue transplantation research. See Bopp, James, Jr.

326. "Charity and Co-Operation," in Davis, Henry.

327. Cataldo, Peter J., and Albert S. Moraczewski. M. Cathleen Kaveny offers a review of the literature and a new approach in her article "Appropriation of Evil: Cooperation's Mirror Image."

328. Smith, Russell E.

329. Miller, L. G.

330. In my view, Fletcher, John C., p. E-17 somewhat misstates the issue when he maintains that "in moral terms, the major difference [between EG and ES cell research] is that [in EG stem cell research] the abortion causes the death of the fetus,

and [in ES research] the research causes the death of the embryo." It is not research that causes the death of the embryo in ES cell research, but the infertility clinician's carrying out of the progenitors' wishes that the embryo be destroyed. The possibility of research only shapes the *manner* in which the embryo's death is carried out.

331. Ibrahim, Youssef M.

332. Bettelheim, Adriel.

333. Nicholas, Wade, (1999).

334. Richard Doerflinger has used NBAC's rejection of the use-derivation distinction to support his criticism of proposed NIH funding guidelines. See Doerflinger, Richard (1999a), 142.

335. Rawls, John (1993), pp. 67, 137–139, 212–254, (1999), p. 155.

336. Gutmann, Amy and Dennis Thompson, p. 89.

337. Warren, Mary Anne, (1997), pp. 170–172, identifies what she calls the "Principle of Transitivity of Respect." This requires us "to the extent that is feasible and morally acceptable . . . to seek to avoid harming entities to which other persons ascribe a high moral status." A similar consideration appears to underlie the "incremental" approach to stem cell research recommended by Fletcher, John C.

338. This does not rule out the creation of federal guidelines to protect the donors of the embryos eventually used in research. Such protections are spelled out in the "Draft National Institutes of Health Guidelines for Research Involving Human Pluripotent Stem Cells (December 1999)."

339. National Bioethics Advisory Commission (1999), pp. v, 19–20, and 58–59.

340. Ibid., pp. iv, 58.

341. Hall, Stephen S.

342. Chapman, Audrey R., Mark S. Frankel, and Michele S. Garfinkle.

343. Doerflinger, Richard M. (1999b).

344. Recent studies suggest that adult stem cells are far less differentiated than was previously believed. Nevertheless, ES cells still appear to be more promising as a source of transplant material. See Vogel, Gretchen (1999).

345. Statement to NBAC, 3 February 1999, National Bioethics Advisory Commission (1999), p. 19.

346. Doerflinger, Richard (1999a), 142. Doerflinger's important role in leading the opposition to federal funding for stem cell research is described by Allen, Arthur.

347. Dworkin, Ronald.

348. Ibid., pp. 11, 90.

349. National Bioethics Advisory Commission (1999), p. 52.

350. Statement of Christopher Currie, 25 August 1999.

351. National Bioethics Advisory Commission (1999), p. iv.

352. Drawing on a single 1993 study, the NBAC report repeatedly affirms that there is a limit to how long a stem cell line can be cultured without undergoing genetic changes (*ibid.*, pp. v, 19–20, 58–59). Scientists on the AAAS working group disputed this claim. The final report also includes a long footnote by Commissioner Alexander Capron (p. 59) seeking to further ground the report's ultimate rejection of the use-vs.-derivation distinction. Capron argues that, in the absence of an explicit federal law banning the creation of embryos for research, excluding the government from involvement in the derivation process would hinder its ability to bar the use of stem cell lines derived from research embryos. Like the scientific arguments, however, this seems a tenuous basis for NBAC's position. Based on the advice of an ethics review panel, NIH is presumably free to impose any ethical restrictions it wishes on

the lines whose use it funds. Furthermore, a ban on lines derived from research embryos could easily be justified in terms of President Clinton's December 1994 executive order prohibiting funding for the creation of research embryos. I suspect that all these arguments were after-the-fact rationalizations aimed at justifying some commissioners' moral discomfort with the use-vs.-derivation distinction.

353. Solter, Davor, and John Gearhart.

354. National Bioethics Advisory Commission (1999), p. 55.

355. The principal issue advanced by the report is the familiar but vague concern over "instrumentalization" of human life. What the report does not address, however, is why the creation of embryos for research for lifesaving purposes (which the report has already maintained is a reason for using spare embryos) raises the question of instrumentalization, while a couple's creation of many more embryos than they need does not. National Bioethics Advisory Commission (1999), p. 56.

356. Fletcher, John C., p. E-13.

357. Ibid.

358. "National Institutes of Health Guidelines for Research Using Human Pluripotent Stem Cells," (Effective August 25, 2000), 65 *Federal Register* 51976. These are also available at the NIH website: http://www.nih.gov/news/stemcell/stemcellguidelines.htm.

359. *New York Times,* 23 August 2000.

360. 106th Congress, S. 2015, "Stem Cell Research Act of 2000."

361. Bettelheim, Adriel; Brainard, Jeffrey; Zitner, Aaron.

362. *Washington Post,* 7 October 1999, p. A34.

Conclusion

363. American Life League, Frequently Asked Questions. Available at http://www.all.org/policy3.htm.

364. Pellegrino, Edmund D., states (p. F-4) "There is no moral or legal basis for subjecting any member of the human species to harm or death in nontherapeutic research based on the prediction that it will die anyway, no matter how certain that prediction may be."

365. The overwhelming majority of negative letters received by the NIH during its comment period on proposed human stem cell research guidelines reflect the Roman Catholic position on this issue established by the National Conference of Catholic Bishops (personal communication from an official of the NIH Office of Science Policy, 21 February 2000).

366. Andrews, Lori B., pp. 303–304.

367. Fletcher, John C., appears to espouse this view when he states that "[f]ederal and state government may also use denial of funding to ameliorate the divisiveness of intractable moral disputes like abortion. Such actions are more understandable in a nation with sharply divided (public and private) systems of health care and research" (p. E-12).

368. Gutmann, Amy, and Dennis Thompson explicitly argue that such access cannot be a matter of majority rule but pertains to basic liberties governed by constitutional rights, pp. 30–31.

369. "The Idea of Public Reason" in Rawls, John (1993), pp. 212–254.

370. Epstein, Steven, pp. 225, 284–285.

371. Rawls notes that citizens and legislators may allowably vote on the basis of religious views when "constitutional essentials and basic justice" are not at issue. See Rawls, John (1993), p. 235. I am arguing that funding priorities for life-saving research involve a matter of "basic justice." I note that Rawls argues that public reason, proceeding from the undeniable value of women's equality, affirms, despite religious objections, that a woman has a right to abortion during the first trimester of a pregnancy (*ibid.*, p. 243). Many of the research-related issues I discuss have no less impact on the equality and health of women than does the right to abortion. I should add, however, that in his more recent *The Law of Peoples,* p. 169, note. 80 Rawls describes this previous mention of abortion as only an illustration of an appropriate mode of reasoning and not yet a "reasonable argument" for such a right. Nevertheless, in this same volume Rawls affirms, correctly in my opinion, that "If we say the gender system includes whatever social arrangements adversely affect the equal basic liberties and opportunities of women, as well as those of their children as future citizens, then surely that system is subject to critique by the principles of justice" (p. 163). Surely basic reproductive health care policy forms a part of a society's gender system in this sense.

372. Mauron, Alex, "The Human Embryo and the Relativity of Biological Individuality."

373. For a fuller account of Jain belief and practice, see Jaini, Padmanab S.

374. Mauron, Alex, p. 67.

375. The same conclusion follows from Mary Anne Warren's "Principle of the Transitivity of Respect," *Moral Status,* pp. 177–172. Although this requires us to "to seek to avoid harming entities to which other persons ascribe a high moral status," it also entitles us "to reject attributions of moral status" that are incompatible with the moral rights of human beings.

376. Rawls, John (1993), p. 217.

377. Lanza et al. (2000b).

378. "Stem Cell Research: Medical Progress with Responsibility: A Report from the Chief Medical Officer's Expert Group Reviewing the Potential of Developments in Stem Cell Research and Cell Nuclear Replacement to Benefit Human Health," Department of Health, June 2000. Available at http://www.doh.gov.uk/cegc/stemcell report.htm.

379. George Jones, "MPs Vote for Research on Human Embryos," *Electronic Telegraph* (The Telegraph online), 20 December 2000. Available at: http://www.telegraph.co.uk:80/et?ac = 001432256857616&rtmo = lvSwuobt&atmo = 99999999&pg = / et/00/12/20/nclon20.html; "UK Enters the Clone Age, BBC News Online, 23 January 2001. Availabile at http://news.bbc.co.uk/hi/english/uk_politics/newsid_1132000/ 1132034.stm.

380. National Institutes of Health Guidelines for Research Using Human Pluripotent Stem Cells, (Effective August 25, 2000), 65 *Federal Register* 51976. These are also available at the NIH website: http://www.nih.gov/news/stemcell/stemcellguidelines.htm.

381. Stolberg, Sheryl Gay, "Stem Cell Research Advocates in Limbo," *New York Times* (online edition), 20 January 2001. Available at: http://www.nytimes.com/ 2001/01/20/health/20STEM.html.

BIBLIOGRAPHY

Abma, J. C. et al. "Fertility, Family Planning, and Women's Health: New Data from the 1995 National Survey of Family Growth." *Vital and Health Statistics* 23/19 (1997), 1–125.

Alfa, Michelle J., Jeffrey J. Sisler, and Godfrey K. M. Harding. "Mycobacterium Abscessus Infection of a Norplant Contraceptive Implant Site." *Canadian Medical Association Journal* 153/9 (1 Nov 1995), 1293–1296.

Allen, Arthur. "God and Science," *Washington Post* (magazine), 15 October 2000, pp. W08FF.

Andrews, Lori B. "State Regulation of Embryo Research." In National Institutes of Health, *Papers Commissioned for the Human Embryo Research Panel*, NIH Publication Number 95-3916 (Bethesda, MD: National Institutes of Health, 1994), vol. 2, pp. 297–407.

Andrews, Lori, and Nanette Elster. "Cross-Cultural Analysis of Policies Regarding Embryo Research." In National Institutes of Health, *Papers Commissioned for the Human Embryo Research Panel*, NIH Publication Number 95-3916 (Bethesda, MD: National Institutes of Health, 1994), vol. 2, pp. 51–296.

Annas, George, Arthur Caplan, and Sherman Elias. "The Politics of Human-Embryo Research—Avoiding Ethical Gridlock." *New England Journal of Medicine* 334/20 (16 May 1996), 1329–1332.

Austin, C. R. *Human Embryos: The Debate on Assisted Reproduction*. Oxford: Oxford University Press, 1989.

Barada, James. "Sexual Function Is a Vital Part of Health." *Business and Health* 16/6 (1998), 55–56.

Benjamin, Martin. "The Value of Consensus." In R. E. Bulger, E. M. Bobby, and H. F. Fineberg, eds., *Society's Choices: Social and Ethical Decision Making in Biomedicine* (Washington, DC: National Academy Press, 1995), pp. 241–260.

Bernasko, J., L. Lynch, R. Lapinski, and R. L. Berkowitz. "Twin Pregnancies Conceived by Assisted Reproductive Techniques: Maternal and Neonatal Outcomes." *Obstetrics and Gynecology* 89/3 (1997), 368–372.

Bernat, James. *Ethical Issues in Neurology* (Boston: Butterworth-Heinemann, 1994).

Bettelheim, Adriel. "Senate Argues Promise and Peril of Human Stem Cell Research." *CQ Weekly*, 19 February 2000, 357–359.

Bigelow, John, and Robert Pargetter. "Morality, Potential Persons, and Abortion." *American Philosophical Quarterly* 25/2 (1988), 173–181.

Biggers, J. D. "In Vitro Fertilization, Embryo Culture and Embryo Transfer in the

Human." In Appendix to Report of the Ethics Advisory Board, *HEW Support of Research Involving Human* In Vitro *Fertilization and Embryo Transfer* (Washington: Government Printing Office 4 May 1979), section 8, pp. 1–50.

Blank, R. H. "Assisted Reproduction and Reproductive Rights: The Case of In Vitro Fertilization." *Politics & the Life Sciences* 16 (1997), 279–288.

Bobik, J. "Soul, Human: 4. Philosophic Analysis." *New Catholic Encyclopedia* (New York: McGraw Hill, 1967–1979), vol. 13, pp. 459–462.

Bok, Sissela. "Ethical Problems of Abortion." *Hastings Center Studies* 2/1 (January 1974), 39–42.

Bonaccorsi, A. C., et al. "Genetic Disorders in Normally Androgenized Infertile Men and the Use of Intracytoplasmic Sperm Injection as a Way of Treatment." *Fertility and Sterility* 67 (1997), 928–931.

Bonduelle, M., et al. "Prospective Follow-Up Study of 423 Children Born after Intracytoplasmic Sperm Injection." *Human Reproduction* 11/7 (1996), 1558–1564.

Bonnicksen, Andrea L. "Creating a Clone in Ninety Days: In Search of a Cloning Policy." *Jurimetrics* 38 (February 1997), 23–31.

Bopp, James, Jr. "Fetal Tissue Transplantation and Moral Complicity with Induced Abortion." In Peter J. Cataldo and Albert S. Moraczewski, eds., *The Fetal Tissue Issue: Medical and Ethical Aspects*, (Braintree, MA: Pope John Center, 1994), pp. 61–69.

Brainard, Jeffrey. "20 Senators Ask NIH Not to Finance Stem Cell Research." *The Chronicle of Higher Education*, 25 February 2000, A40.

Brent, R. L. "The Magnitude of Congenital Malformations." In M. Marois, ed., *Prevention of Physical and Mental Congenital Defects: Proceedings of the International Conference Held in Strasbourg, France, 10–17 October, 1982: Part A. The Scope of the Problem*. Series, *Progress in Clinical and Biological Research*, 163a (New York: Alan R. Liss, 1985), pp. 55–68.

Bristow, Robert E., and Beth Y. Karlan. "Ovulation Induction, Infertility, and Ovarian Cancer Risk." *Fertility and Sterility* 66/4 (1996), 499–507.

Brock, Dan W. "The Non-Identity Problem and Genetic Harms—The Case of Wrongful Handicaps." *Bioethic*, 9 (1995a), 269–275.

Brock, Dan W. "Public Moral Discourse." In Ruth E. Bulger, Elizabeth M. Bobby, and Harvey V. Fineberg, eds., *Society's Choices: Social and Ethical Decision Making in Biomedicine* (Washington, DC: National Academy Press, 1995b), pp. 215–240.

Brock, Dan W. "Funding New Reproductive Technologies: Should They Be Included in Health Insurance Benefit Packages?" In Cynthia B. Cohen, ed., *New Ways of Making Babies: The Case of Egg Donation* (Bloomington: Indiana University Press, 1996), pp. 213–227.

Brock, Dan W. "Reproductive Freedom and the Prevention of Harm." In Allen Buchanan, Dan W. Brock, Norman Daniels, and Daniel Wikler, *From Chance to Choice: Genetics and Justice* (Cambridge: Cambridge University Press, 2000), pp. 204–257.

Brody, Baruch. *Abortion and the Sanctity of Human Life* (Cambridge, MA: MIT Press, 1975).

Buckle, Stephen. "Arguing from Potential." In Peter Singer et al., eds., *Embryo Experimentation: Ethical, Legal and Social Issues* (Cambridge: Cambridge University Press, 1990), pp. 93–108.

Buckle, Stephen, Karen Dawson, and Peter Singer. "The Syngamy Debate: When Precisely Does a Human Life Begin." In Peter Singer et al., eds., *Embryo Experi-*

mentation: Ethical Legal and Social Issues (Cambridge: Cambridge University Press, 1990), pp. 213–225.

Bulmer, M. G. *The Biology of Twinning in Man* (Oxford: Clarendon Press, 1970).

Burgess, J. A., and S. A. Tawia. "When Did You First Begin to Feel It—Locating the Beginning of Human Consciousness." *Bioethics* 10/1 (1966), 1–26.

Callahan, Daniel. "The Puzzle of Profound Respect." *Hastings Center Report* 25/1 (1995), 39–40.

Campbell, Courtney S. "Commissioned Paper: Religious Perspectives on Human Cloning" (1997). Available at the National Bioethics Advisory Commission Website: http://bioethics.gov/pubs.html.

Campbell, Courtney S. "In Whose Image: Religion and the Controversy of Human Cloning." *Second Opinion*, no. 1, September 1999, 24–43.

Caplan, Arthur L. "The Meaning of the Holocaust for Bioethics." *The Hastings Center Report* 19/4 (1989), 2–3.

Caplan, Arthur L., ed. *When Medicine Went Mad: Bioethics and the Holocaust* (Totowa, NJ: Humana Press, 1992).

Carlson, Bruce M. *Patten's Foundations of Embryology*, 5th ed. (New York: McGraw Hill, 1988).

Carlson, Bruce M. *Human Embryology and Developmental Biology* (St. Louis: Mosby, 1994).

Carmen, Ira H. "Washington Politics and Genetic Engineering Research: When Worlds Collide." *Human Gene Therapy* 7 (1 January 1996), 97–106.

Cataldo, Peter J., and Albert S. Moraczewski, eds. *The Fetal Tissue Issue: Medical and Ethical Aspects*. (Braintree, MA: Pope John Center, 1994).

Centers for Disease Control and Prevention et al. *1995 Assisted Reproductive Technology Success Rates*, vol. 1 (Atlanta: Centers for Disease Control and Prevention, 1997).

Chan, A. W. S., et al. "Clonal Propagation of Primate Offspring by Embryo Splitting." *Science* 287 (14 January 2000), 317–319.

Chapman, Audrey R., Mark S. Frankel, and Michelle S. Garfinkle. *Stem Cell Research and Applications: Monitoring the Frontiers of Biomedical Research* (Washington, DC: American Association for the Advancement of Science and the Institute for Civil Society, 1999).

Charatan, Fred B. "Anatomy Textbook Has Nazi Origins." *British Medical Journal* 313/7070 (1996), 1422.

Charo, Alta. "'La Pénible Valse Hésitation': Fetal Tissue Research Review and the Use of Bioethics Commissions in France and the United States." In R. E. Bulger, E. M. Bobby, and H. F. Fineberg, eds., *Society's Choices: Social and Ethical Decision Making in Biomedicine* (Washington, DC: National Academy Press, 1995a), pp. 477–500.

Charo, Alta. "The Hunting of the Snark: The Moral Status of Embryos, Right-to-Lifers, and Third World Women." *Stanford Law & Policy Review* 6 (1995b), 11–27.

Charo, Alta. "Dealing with Dolly: Cloning and the National Bioethics Advisory Commission." *Jurimetrics* 38 (February 1997), 11–22.

Chief Medical Officer's Expert Group. "Stem Cell Research: Medical Progress with Responsibility: A Report from the Chief Medical Officer's Expert Group Reviewing the Potential of Developments in Stem Cell Research and Cell Nuclear Replacement to Benefit Human Health," Department of Health, June 2000. Available at http://www.doh.gov.uk/cegc/stemcellreport.htm.

Childress, James F. "A Response to Ronald Green 'Conferred Rights and the Fetus'." *Journal of Religious Ethics* 2/1 (1974), 77–83.

CIBA Foundation. *Human Embryo Research: Yes or No* (Tavistock Publications, London, 1986).

Cohen, Cynthia B. "'Give Me Children or I Shall Die!': New Reproductive Technologies and Harm to Children." *Hastings Center Report*, 26/2 (1996), 19–27.

Cole-Turner, Ronald, ed. *Human Cloning: Religious Responses* (Louisville, Kentucky: Westminster John Knox Press, 1997).

Consultants to the Advisory Committee to the Director, National Institutes of Health. *Report of the Human Fetal Tissue Transplantation Research Panel*, December 1988.

Cook-Deegan, Robert. *The Gene Wars: Science, Politics, and the Human Genome* (New York: W. W. Norton, 1994).

Corea, Gena. *The Mother Machine: Reproductive Technologies from Artificial Insemination to Artificial Wombs* (New York: Harper & Row, 1985).

Council of Europe. *Convention for the Protection of Human Rights and Dignity of the Human Being with Regard to the Application of Biology and Medicine, Convention on Human Rights and Medicine* (Strasbourg: Directorate of Legal Affairs, 1996).

Crosby, U. D., B. E. Schwartz, K. L. Gluck, and S. F. Heartwell. "A Preliminary Report of Norplant Insertions in a Large Urban Family Planning Program." *Contraception* 48 (1993), 359–366.

Culver, Charles, and Bernard Gert. *Philosophy in Medicine* (Oxford University Press, New York, 1982).

Davis, Dena S. "Genetic Dilemmas and the Child's Right to an Open Future." *Rutgers Law Journal* 28 (1997), 549–592.

Davis, Henry. *Moral and Pastoral Theology*, 8th ed., vol. 1 (London: Sheed and Ward, 1959).

Delaney, Joseph F. "Death." *The Catholic Encyclopedia* (1908), vol. 4, pp. 660–663.

Diamond, James. "Abortion, Animation, and Biological Humanization," *Theological Studies* 36 (1975), 305–324.

Doerflinger, Richard. "The Ethics of Funding Embryonic Stem Cell Research: A Catholic Viewpoint." *Kennedy Institute of Ethics Journal* 9/2 (1999a), 137–150.

Doerflinger, Richard. "Testimony of Richard M. Doerflinger on Behalf of the Committee for Pro-Life Activities of the National Conference of Catholic Bishops Before the Senate Appropriations Subcommittee on Labor, Health and Education, Hearing on Legal Status of Embryonic Stem Cell Research, 26 January 1999" (1999b).

Dolan, Edwin G. *TANSTAAFL: The Economic Strategy for Environmental Crisis* (New York: Holt, Rinehart and Winston, 1971).

Donceel, Joseph. "Immediate Animation and Delayed Hominization." *Theological Studies* 31 (1970), 76–105.

Donchin, Anne. "Procreation, Power and Subjectivity: Feminist Approaches to New Reproductive Technologies." Wellesley College Center for Research on Women, Wellesley, MA, Working Paper Series No. 260, pp. 1–22.

Dworkin, Ronald. *Life's Dominion: An Argument About Abortion, Euthanasia, and Individual Freedom* (New York: Knopf, 1993).

Edwards, Robert, and Patrick Steptoe. *A Matter of Life* (New York: William Morrow and Company, 1980).

Englert, Yvon. "The Fate of Supernumerary Embryos: What Do Patients Think about It?" In Elisabeth Hildt and Dietmar Mieth, eds., *In Vitro Fertilization in the*

1990s: Towards a Medical, Social, and Ethical Evaluation (Aldershot: Ashgate, 1999), pp. 227–232.

Epstein, Steven. *Impure Science: AIDS, Activism, and the Politics of Knowledge* (Berkeley: University of California Press, 1996).

Ethics Advisory Board, Department of Health, Education and Welfare. "Report and Conclusions: HEW Support of Research Involving Human In Vitro Fertilization and Embryo Transfer." 4 May 1979, Federal Register 44, no. 118, Monday, 18 June 1979.

Evans, Donald, ed. *Conceiving the Embryo: Ethics, Law and Practice in Human Embryology* (The Hague: Martinus Nijhoff, 1996).

Feinberg, Joel. "The Child's Right to an Open Future." In W. Aiken and H. LaFollett, eds., *Whose Child? Children's Rights, Parental Authority and State Power* (Totowa, NJ: Rowman and Littlefield, 1980), pp. 124–153.

Feinberg, Joel. "Wrongful Life and the Counterfactual Element in Harming." In *Freedom and Fulfillment: Philosophical Essays* (Princeton, Princeton University Press, 1992), pp. 3–36.

Fleck, Leonard M. "Abortion, Deformed Fetuses, and the Omega Pill." *Philosophical Studies* 36/3 (October 1979), 271–283.

Fletcher, John. "Deliberating Incrementally on Human Pluripotential Stem Cell Research." In National Bioethics Advisory Commission, *Ethical Issues in Human Stem Cell Research, Vol. II, Commissioned Papers* (Rockville, MD: National Bioethics Advisory Commission, January 1999), pp. E1–E50. Also available at the NBAC Website: http://bioethics.gov/pubs.html.

Ford, Norman M. *When Did I Begin?* (Cambridge, Cambridge University Press, 1988).

Fortes, Meyer. *Religion, Morality and the Person: Essays on Tallensi Religion* (Cambridge: Cambridge University Press, 1987).

Fotion, Nick, and Jan C. Heller. *Contingent Future Persons* (Dordrecht: Kluwer Academic Publishers, 1997).

Freed, C. R., B. R. Breeze, and S. A. Schenck. "Transplantation of Fetal Mesencephalic Tissue in Parkinson's Disease." *New England Journal of Medicine* 333/11(1995), 730–731.

French, Howard W. "In Africa's Back-Street Clinics, Illicit Abortions Take a Heavy Toll," *New York Times*, Wednesday, 3 June 1998, pp. A1, A3.

Friedler, S., S. Mashiach, and N. Laufer. "Births in Israel Resulting from In-Vitro Fertilization/Embryo Transfer; 1982–1989: National Registry of the Israeli Association for Fertility Research." *Human Reproduction* 7 (1992), 1159–1163.

Fuller, Paul N. "Malignant Melanoma of the Ovary and Exposure to Clomiphene Citrate: A Case Report and Review of the Literature." *American Journal of Obstetrics and Gynecology* 180/6, part 1 (1999), 1499–1503.

Galjaard, H., ed. *Aspects of Genetic Disease* (Basel, Switzerland: Karger, 1984).

Geron Ethics Advisory Board. "Research with Human Embryonic Stem Cells: Ethical Considerations." *Hastings Center Report* 29/2 (1999), 31–36.

Goldberg, Carey. "Web Site Selling Models' Eggs." *The Gazette* (Montreal) 23 October 1999, p. D19.

Gray, Bradford H. "Bioethics Commissions: What Can We Learn from Past Successes and Failures." In Ruth E. Bulger, Elizabeth M. Bobby, and Harvey V. Fineberg, eds., *Society's Choices: Social and Ethical Decision Making in Biomedicine* (Washington, DC: National Academy Press, 1995), pp. 261–306.

Green, Ronald M. "Abortion and Promise-Keeping." *Christianity and Crisis*, 27/8 (15 May 1967), 109–113.

Green, Ronald M. "Conferred Rights and the Fetus." *Journal of Religious Ethics*, 2/1 (Spring 1974), 55–75.

Green, Ronald M. "Health Care and Justice in Contract Theory Perspective." In Robert Veatch and Roy Branson, eds., *Ethics and Health Policy* (Cambridge, MA: Ballinger Books, 1976a), pp. 111–126.

Green, Ronald M. *Population Growth and Justice: An Examination of Moral Issues Raised by Rapid Population Growth* (Scholars Press: Missoula, MT, 1976b).

Green, Ronald M. "Toward a Copernican Revolution in Our Thinking about Life's Beginning and Life's End." *Soundings* 66/2 (Summer 1983), 152–173.

Green, Ronald M. "The Irrelevance of Theology for Sexual Ethics." In Earl Shelp, ed., *Sexuality and Medicine, Vol. II: Ethical Viewpoints in Transition* (Dordrecht: D. Reidel, 1987), pp. 249–270.

Green, Ronald M. *Religion and Moral Reason* (New York: Oxford University Press, 1988).

Green, Ronald M. "The Challenge of Controlling Costs as We Expand Health Care Access." *Second Opinion* 19/4 (April 1994a), 64–67.

Green, Ronald M. *The Ethical Manager* (New York: Macmillan, 1994b).

Green, Ronald M. "Jewish Teaching on the Sanctity and Quality of Life." In Edmund D. Pellegrino and Alan I. Faden, eds., *Jewish and Catholic Bioethics: An Ecumenical Dialogue* (Washington, DC: Georgetown University Press, 1998), pp. 25–42.

Green, Ronald M. "Jewish and Christian Ethics: What Can We Learn from One Another?" (Presidential Address to the Society of Christian Ethics, 1998). In *The Annual of the Society of Christian Ethics* (Washington, DC: Georgetown University Press, 1999a), pp. 1–16.

Green, Ronald M. "Religion and Bioethics." In Dena S. Davis and Laurie Zoloth-Dorfman, eds., *Notes from a Narrow Ridge* (Frederick, MD: University Publishing Group, 1999b), pp. 165–181.

Green, Ronald M., Bernard Gert, and K. Danner Clouser. "The Method of Public Morality versus the Method of Principlism." *The Journal of Medicine and Philosophy* 18 (1993), 477–489.

Green, Ronald M. "What Does it Mean to Treat Someone as a 'Means Only'?" *Kennedy Institute of Ethics Journal* (2001). In press.

Gutmann, Amy, and Dennis Thompson. *Democracy and Disagreement.* (Cambridge, MA: Belknap Press, 1996).

Hall, Stephen S. "The Recycled Generation." *New York Times Magazine*, Sunday, 30 January 2000, pp. 30ff.

Hanser, M. "Harming Future People." *Philosophy and Public Affairs* 19 (1990), 47–70.

Hanson, Michele A., and Daniel A. Dumesic. "Initial Evaluation and Treatment of Infertility in a Primary-Care Setting." *Mayo Clinic Proceedings* 73/7 (1998), 681–685.

Hardacre, Helen. *Marketing the Menacing Fetus in Japan* (Berkeley: University of California Press, 1997).

Hare, R. M. "Public Policy in a Pluralist Society." In Peter Singer et al., eds., *Embryo Experimentation: Ethical, Legal and Social Issues* (Cambridge: Cambridge University Press, 1990), pp. 183–194.

Harper, J. C., and A. H. Handyside. "The Current Status of Preimplantation Genetic Diagnosis." *Current Obstetrics and Gynecology* 4 (1994), 143–149.

Hellegers, André. "Fetal development." *Theological Studies* 31 (1970), 3–9.

Heller, J. C., ed., *Human Genome Research & The Challenge of Contingent Future Persons* (Omaha: Creighton University Press, 1996).

Herbst, A. L. et al. "A Comparison of Pregnancy Experience in DES-Exposed and DES-Unexposed Daughters." *Journal of Reproductive Medicine* 24 (1980), 62–69.

Heyd, David. *Genethics: Moral Issues in the Creation of People* (Berkeley: University of California Press, 1992).

Hogan, Brigid. "Lesch-Nyhan Syndrome. Engineering Mutant Mice [News]." *Nature* 326/6110 (1987), 240–241.

Horovitz, Bruce. "Selling Beautiful Babies." *USA Today* 25 October 1999, p. 1A.

Human Fertilisation and Embryology Authority. *Code of Practice* (1998), 4th ed., July 1998. Available at the HFEA website: http://www.hfea.gov.uk/frame.htm.

Huxley, Aldous. *Brave New World* (London: Chatto & Windus, 1932).

Ibrahim, Youssef M. "Ethical Furor Erupts in Britain: Should Embryos Be Destroyed?" *New York Times,* 1 August 1996, late ed., p. A1.

Jackson, Anthony. "Wrongful Life and Wrongful Birth: The English Conception." *The Journal of Legal Medicine* 17 (1996), 349–381.

Jaini, Padmanab S. *The Jaina Path of Purification* (Berkeley: University of California Press, 1979).

Jecker, N. S. "The Ascription of Rights in Wrongful Life Suits." *Law and Philosophy* 6 (1987), 149–165.

Jos, P. H., M. F. Marshall, and M. Perlmutter. "The Charleston Policy on Cocaine Use During Pregnancy: A Cautionary Tale." *Journal of Law, Medicine & Ethics* 23 (1995), 120–128.

Kahn, Axel. "L'Acharnement Procréatif." *Le Monde,* 16 March 1999, p. 13.

Kahn, Jeffrey P. "A Temporary Halt: National Bioethics Commissions and NBAC's Cloning Report." *Jurimetrics* 38 (February 1997), 33–34.

Kant, Immanuel. *Foundation of the Metaphysics of Morals,* tr. Lewis White Beck (Indianapolis: Library of Liberal Arts, 1959).

Kass, Leon R. "Babies by Means of In Vitro Fertilization: Unethical Experiments on the Unborn." *New England Journal of Medicine* 285 (1971), 1174–1179.

Katz, Jeffrey L. "After Noisy Debate, Panel Keeps Family Planning Services Law." *Congressional Quarterly* (29 June 1996), 1874–1876.

Kaveny, M. Cathleen. "Appropriation of Evil: Cooperation's Mirror Image." *Theological Studies* 61(2000), 280–313.

Kelly, M. B. "The Rightful Position in 'Wrongful Life' Actions." *Hasting Law Journal* 42 (1991), 505–589.

Kleiman, Dena. "Anguished Search to Cure Infertility." *The New York Times Magazine,* 16 December 1979, pp. 38ff.

Koch, Lene. "Two Decades of IVF: A Critical Appraisal." In Elizabeth Hildt and Dietmar Mieth, eds., *In Vitro Fertilization in the 1990s: Towards a Medical, Social, and Ethical Evaluation* (Aldershot: Ashgate, 1999), pp. 19–31.

Kolata, Gina. "Scientist Clones Embryos, and Creates an Ethical Challenge." *New York Times,* 24 October 1993, p. A1.

Kolata, Gina. "Little-Known Panel Challenged to Make Quick Cloning Study." *New York Times,* 18 March 1997a, p. C9.

Kolata, Gina. "Successful Births Reported with Frozen Human Eggs." *New York Times,* 17 October 1997b, pp. A1, A16.

Kolata, Gina. *Clone: The Road to Dolly and the Path Ahead* (New York: William Morrow and Company, 1998).

Kolata, Gina. "When a Cell Does an Embryo's Work, a Debate Is Born." *New York Times,* 9 February 1999a, p. C2.

Kolata, Gina. "Scientists Place Jellyfish Genes into Monkeys." *New York Times,* 23 December 1999b, p. A1.

Kordower, J. H. et al., "Neuropathological Evidence of Graft Survival and Striatal Reinnervation after the Transplantation of Fetal Mesencephalic Tissue in a Patient with Parkinson's Disease." *New England Journal of Medicine* 332/17 (1995), 1118–1124.

Kovács, Jósef. "The Idea of Brain Birth in Connection with the Moral Status of the Embryo and Foetus." In Donald Evans, ed., *Conceiving the Embryo: Ethics, Law and Practice in Human Embryology* (The Hague; Martinus Nijhoff, 1996), pp. 221–245.

Kuhse, Helga, and Peter Singer. "Individuals, Humans and Personhood: The Issue of Moral Status," in Peter Singer et al., eds., *Embryo Experimentation: Ethical, Legal and Social Issues* (Cambridge: Cambridge University Press, 1990), pp. 65–75.

Kurinczuk, J. J., and C. Bower. "Birth Defects in Infants Conceived by Intracytoplasmic Sperm Injection: An Alternative Interpretation." *British Medical Journal* (1997), 1260–1265.

Labosky, P. A., D. P. Barlow, and B. L. Hogan. "Embryonic Germ Cell Lines and Their Derivation from Mouse Primordial Germ Cells." *Ciba Foundation Symposium* 182 (1994), 157–168 (discussion 168–178).

Lafleur, William R. *Liquid Life: Abortion and Buddhism in Japan* (Princeton, NJ: Princeton University Press, 1992).

Lanza, Robert P., Jose P. Cibelli, and Michael D. West. "Commentary: Human Therapeutic Cloning." *Nature Medicine* 5/9 (September 1999), 975–977.

Lanza R. P. et al. "Extension of Cell Life-Span and Telomere Length in Animals Cloned from Senescent Somatic Cells." *Science* 288 (28 April 2000a), 665–669.

Lanza R. P. et al. "The Ethical Validity of Using Nuclear Transfer In Human Transplantation." *Journal of the American Medical Association* 284/24 (27 December 2000b), 3175–3179.

Larsen, William J. *Human Embryology* (New York: Churchill Livingstone, 1997).

Lauritzen, Paul. *Pursuing Parenthood: Ethical Issues in Assisted Reproduction* (Bloomington, Indiana: Indiana University Press, 1993).

Lauritzen, Paul. *Cloning and The Future of Embryo Research* (New York: Oxford University Press, 2001).

Lebacqz, Karen. "Feminism and Bioethics: An Overview." *Second Opinion* 17/2 (1991), 11–25.

LeJeune, Jerome. *The Concentration Can* (San Francisco: Ignatius, 1992).

Lewontin, Richard. "The Confusion over Cloning." *New York Review of Books,* 23 October 1997, pp. 18ff. www.nybooks.com/nyrev/WWWarchdisplay.cgi? 1997102318R.

Liebmann-Smith, Joan. *In Pursuit of Pregnancy* (New York: Newmarket Press, 1987).

Locke, John. *An Essay Concerning Human Understanding,* A. D. Woozley, ed. (Cleveland, OH: World, 1964).

Lockwood, Michael. "When Does a Life Begin?" In Michael Lockwood, ed., *Moral Dilemmas in Modern Medicine* (London: Oxford University Press, 1985), pp. 9–31.

Lockwood, Michael. "Human Identity and the Primitive Streak." *Hastings Center Report* 25/1 (1995), 45.

Macklin, Ruth. "Reproductive Technologies in Developing Countries." *Bioethics* 9/3-4 (1995), 276–282.

Maranto, Gina. "Embryo Overpopulation." *Scientific American* 274/4 (1996), 12, 16.

Marquis, Don. "Why Abortion is Immoral." *Journal of Philosophy* 86/4 (1989), 183–202.

Marshall, Eliot. "Rules on Human Embryo Research Due Out," *Science* 265 (19 August 1994), 1024–26.

Marshall, Eliot. "A Versatile Cell Line Raises Scientific Hopes, Legal Questions." *Science* 282 (6 November 1998), 1014–1015.

Martin, Gwen. "Selling My Eggs." *Glamour Magazine,* May 1994, 168.

Mason, Mary Martin. *The Miracle Seekers: An Anthology of Infertility* (Indianapolis: Perspectives Press, 1987).

Massey, J. B., M. J. Tucker, H. J. Malter, and J. L. Hall. "Blastomere Separation: Potential for Human Investigation." *Assisted Reproduction Reviews* 4 (1994), 50–59.

Matsui, Y. et al. "Effect of Steel Factor and Leukaemia Inhibitory Factor on Murine Primordial Germ Cells in Culture." *Nature* 353/6346 (1991), 750–752.

Mauron, Alex. "The Human Embryo and the Relativity of Biological Individuality." In Donald Evans, ed., *Conceiving the Embryo: Ethics, Law and Practice in Human Embryology* (The Hague: Martinus Nijhoff, 1996), pp. 55–74.

McCormick, Richard A. "Who or What is the Pre-Embryo?" *Kennedy Institute of Ethics Journal* 1 (1991), 1–15.

Miller, L. G. "Scandal." *New Catholic Encyclopedia* (New York: McGraw Hill, 1967), vol. 12, pp. 1112–1113.

Moe, Kristine. "Should the Nazi Research Data Be Cited?" *The Hastings Center Report* 14/6 (1984), 5–7.

Moore, Keith L., and T. V. N. Persaud. *The Developing Human: Clinically Oriented Embryology*, 6th ed. (Philadelphia: W. B. Saunders, 1998).

Moraczewski, Albert S. "Is the Biological Subject of Human Rights Present from Conception." In Peter J. Cataldo and Albert S. Moraczewski, eds., *The Fetal Tissue Issue: Medical and Ethical Aspects* (Braintree, MA: Pope John Center, 1994), pp. 33–59.

Morison, Robert. "Death: Process or Event?" *Science* 173 (20 August 1971), 694–698.

Morrow, David J. "Maker of Norplant Offers a Settlement in Suit over Side Effects." *New York Times,* 27 August 1999, p. A1.

Müller, Hansjakob. "Connecting Lines from a Medical Point of View." In Elisabeth Hildt and Dietmar Mieth, eds., *In Vitro Fertilization in the 1990s: Towards a Medical, Social, and Ethical Evaluation* (Aldershot: Ashgate, 1999), pp. 281–291.

Nagy, András et al. "Derivation of Completely Cell Culture-Derived Mice from Early-Passage Embryonic Stem Cells." *Proceedings of the National Academy of Sciences* 90 (September 1993), 8424–8428.

Narveson, Jan. "Future People and Us." In R. I. Sikora and B. Barry, eds., *Obligations to Future Generations* (Philadelphia: Temple University Press, 1974), pp. 38–60.

National Bioethics Advisory Commission. *Cloning Human Beings: Report and Recommendations of the National Bioethics Advisory Commission* (Rockville, MD, June 1997). Available at http://bioethics.gov/pubs.html.

National Bioethics Advisory Commission. *Ethical Issues in Stem Cell Research, Vol. 1, Report and Recommendations* (National Bioethics Advisory Commission: Rockville, MD, September 1999). Available at http://bioethics.gov/pubs.html.

National Commission for the Protection of Human Subjects of Biomedical and Behavioral Research. *Report and Recommendations: Research on the Fetus* (1975). Reprinted in 40 Fed. Reg. 33, 530 (1976).

National Institutes of Health. *Report of the Human Embryo Research Panel* (Bethesda, MD: National Institutes of Health, September 1994a), vol. 1.

National Institutes of Health. *Papers Commissioned for the Human Embryo Research Panel*. Publication Number 95-3916 (Bethesda, MD: National Institutes of Health, 1994b), vol. 2.

National Institutes of Health Guidelines for Research Using Human Pluripotent Stem Cells, (Effective 25 August 2000). 65 Federal Register 51976. Also available at http://www.nih.gov/news/stemcell/stemcellguidelines.htm.

Nelkin, Dorothy, and Lori Andrews. "Homo Economicus: Commercialization of Body Tissue in the Age of Biotechnology." *Hastings Center Report* 28/5 (1998), 30–39.

Nelson, H. L. "Dethroning Choice: Analogy, Personhood, and the New Reproductive Technologies." *Journal of Law, Medicine, and Ethics* 23 (1995), 129–135.

Neumann, Peter J. et al. "The Cost of a Successful Delivery with In Vitro Fertilization." *New England Journal of Medicine* 331/4 (1994), 239–243.

New York State Task Force on Life and the Law. *Assisted Reproductive Technologies: Analysis and Recommendations for Public Policy* (New York: The New York State Task Force on Life and the Law, 1998).

NIH Revitalization Act of 1993. Pub. L. No 103-43, Sec. 492A (June 10, 1993).

Noonan, John T. *The Morality of Abortion* (Cambridge, MA: Harvard University Press, 1970).

Norman, C. "IVF Moratorium to End?" *Science* 241 (1988), 405.

Olanow, C. W., J. H. Kordower, and T. B. Freeman. "Fetal Nigral Transplantation as a Therapy for Parkinson's Disease." *Trends in Neurosciences* 1/3 (1996), 102–109.

O'Rahilly, Ronan, and Fabiola Müller. *Human Embryology & Teratology* (New York: Wiley-Liss, 1992).

Orentlicher, David. "Cloning and the Preservation of Family Integrity." *Louisiana Law Review* 59/4 (1999), 1019–1040.

Oritz, M. E., and H. Croxatto. "Mode of Action of IUDs." *Contraception* 36 (1987), 37–53.

Osburn, R. A. "Death." *New Catholic Encyclopedia* (1967), vol. 14, pp. 684–685.

Parfit, Derek. *Reasons and Persons* (Oxford: Clarendon Press, 1984).

Paulson, Richard J. "Fertility Drugs and Ovarian Epithelial Cancer: Is There a Link?" *Journal of Assisted Reproduction and Genetics,* 13/10 (1996), 751–756.

Pellegrino, Edmund D. "Testimony of Edmund D. Pellegrino, M.D." In *National Bioethics Advisory Commission (NBAC), Human Stem Cell Research, Volume III Religious Perspectives* (Rockville, MD: National Bioethics Advisory Commission, June 2000), pp. F1–F5.

Pence, Gregory E. *Who's Afraid of Human Cloning?* (Lanham, MD: Rowman & Littlefield, 1998).

Peters, P. G., Jr. "Rethinking Wrongful Life: Bridging the Boundary Between Tort and Family Law." *Tulane Law Review* 67 (1992), 397–454.

Phillips, P. "New Surgical Approaches to Parkinson Disease." *Journal of the American Medical Association* 282/12 (1999), 1117–1118.

Pollack, Andrew. "Small Company Gains High Profile in the Scientific World." *New York Times,* 6 November 1998, p. A24.

Porter, Rebecca. "Insurance Companies Dispute Duty to Reimburse for Viagra." *Trial* 34/8 (1998), 84–85.

Post, Stephen G. "The Echo of Nuremberg: Nazi Data and Ethics." *Journal of Medical Ethics* 17/1 (1991), 42–44.

President's Commission for the Study of Ethical Problems in Medicine and Biomedi-cal and Behavioral Research. *Defining Death: Medical, Legal and Ethical Issues in the Determination of Death* (Washington DC: Government Printing Office, 1981).

Preston, Richard. "Profiles: The Genome Warrior." *The New Yorker*, 12 June 2000, 66–83.

Purdy, L. M. "Genetic Diseases: Can Having Children Be Immoral?" In J. J. Buckley, ed., *Genetics Now: Ethical Issues in Genetic Research* (Washington DC: University Press of America, 1978), pp. 25–39.

Ramsey, Paul. "Shall We 'Reproduce' I. The Medical Ethics of In Vitro Fertilization." *Journal of the American Medical Association* 220/10 (1974), 1346–1350; and II. "Rejoinders and Future Forecasts," *Journal of the American Medical Association* 220/11 (1974), 1480–1485.

Rawls, John. *A Theory of Justice* (Cambridge, MA: Harvard University Press, 1971).

Rawls, John. *Political Liberalism* (New York: Columbia University Press, 1993).

Rawls, John. *The Law of Peoples* (Cambridge, MA: Harvard University Press, 1999).

Raymond, J. G. *Women as Wombs* (San Francisco: Harper, 1993).

Roberts, C. J., and C. R. Lowe. "Where Have all the Conceptions Gone?" *The Lancet* 1 (1 March 1975), 498–499.

Roberts, Melinda. *Child versus Childmaker: Future Persons and Present Duties in Ethics and the Law* (Lanham, MD: Rowman & Littlefield, 1998).

Robertson, John A. *Children of Choice* (Princeton: Princeton University Press, 1994).

Robertson, John A. "Wrongful Life, Federalism, and Procreative Liberty: A Critique of the NBAC Cloning Report." *Jurimetrics* 38 (February 1997), 69–82.

Robertson, John A. "Liberty, Identity, and Human Cloning." *Texas Law Review* 76/6 (May 1998), 1436–1437.

Rossing, Mary Anne et al. "Ovarian Tumors in a Cohort of Infertile Women." *New England Journal of Medicine* 331/12 (1994), 771–776.

Rothenberg, Karen H. "Breast Cancer, the Genetic 'Quick Fix' and the Jewish Com-munity: Ethical, Legal and Social Challenges." *Health Matrix* 7/1 (1997), 98–125.

Rothman, Barbara Katz. *Recreating Motherhood: Ideology and Technology in a Patri-archal Society* (New York: W. W. Norton & Co., 1989).

Royal Commission on New Reproductive Technologies. *Proceed with Care, Report of the Royal Commission on New Reproductive Technologies* (Ottawa, Canada: Minis-ter of Government Services, 1993), 2 vols.

Rubenstein, D. S., D. C. Thomasma, E. A. Schon, M. J. Zinaman. "Germ-Line Ther-apy to Cure Mitochondrial Disease: Protocol and Ethics of In Vitro Ovum Nuclear Transplantation." *Cambridge Quarterly of Healthcare Ethics* 4 (1995), 316–339.

Ryan, Maura A. "Creating Embryos for Research: On Weighing Symbolic Costs." In Paul Lauritzen, ed. *Cloning and the Future of Embryo Research* (New York: Ox-ford University Press, 2001), pp. 50–66.

Sadler, T. W. *Langman's Medical Embryology*, 6th ed. (Baltimore: Williams & Wilkins, 1990).

Sarma, Seshu P., and Robert P. Hatcher. "Gynecology: Neurovascular Injury During Removal of Levonorgestrel Implants." *American Journal of Obstetrics and Gyne-cology* 172/1 (1996), 120–121.

Saunders, K., J. Spensley, J. Munro, and G. Halasz. "Growth and Physical Outcome of Children Conceived by In Vitro Fertilization." *Pediatrics* 97 (1996), 688–692.

Scott, R. T., Jr. et al. "Embryo Quality and Pregnancy Rates in Patients Attempting Pregnancy Through In Vitro Fertilization." *Fertility and Sterility* 55 (1991), 426–428.

Seelye, K. Q. "Clinton Bans Federal Money for Efforts to Clone Humans." *New York Times,* 5 March 1997, p. A13.

Seidelman, William E. "In Memoriam: Medicine's Confrontation with Evil." *The Hastings Center Report* 19/6 (1989), 5.

Seidelman, William E. "Nuremberg Lamentation: For the Forgotten Victims of Medical Science." *British Medical Journal* 313/7070 (1996), 1463–1467.

Shamblot, Michael J. et al. "Derivation of Pluripotential Stem Cells from Cultured Human Primordial Germ Cells." *Proceedings of the National Academy of Sciences* 95 (November 1998), 13,726–13,731.

Shannon, Thomas, and Allan B. Woltor. "Reflections on the Moral Status of the Pre-Embryo." *Theological Studies* 51 (1990), 603–626.

Sheldon, Tony. "European Experts Produce Draft on Bioethics." *British Medical Journal* 309 (23 July 1994), 221.

Shy, K. K. et al. "Genital Tract Examinations and Zona-Free Hamster Egg Penetration Test for Men Exposed in Utero to Diethylstilbestrol." *Fertility and Sterility* 42 (1984), 772–778.

Sidgwick, Henry. *The Methods of Ethics* (New York: Dover Books, 1966).

Siker, Jeffrey S., ed. *Homosexuality in the Church* (Louisville, KY; Westminster John Knox Press, 1994).

Silver, Lee. *Remaking Eden: Cloning and Beyond in a Brave New World* (New York: Avon Books, 1997).

Singer, Peter. *Animal Liberation: A New Ethics for Our Treatment of Animals* (New York: Avon Books, 1975).

Singer, Peter. "A Utilitarian Population Principle." In M. Bayles, ed., *Ethics and Population* (Cambridge, MA: Schenkman Publishing Company, 1976), pp. 81–99.

Singer, Peter. *Practical Ethics* (Cambridge: Cambridge University Press, 1979).

Singer, Peter, and Karen Dawson. "IVF Technology and the Argument from Potential." In Peter Singer et al., eds., *Embryo Experimentation: Ethical, Legal and Social Issues* (Cambridge: Cambridge University Press, 1990), pp. 76–89.

Singer, Peter et al., eds. *Embryo Experimentation: Ethical, Legal and Social Issues* (Cambridge: Cambridge University Press, 1990).

Sivin, I. "IUDs are Contraceptives not Abortifacients." *Studies in Family Planning* 20 (1989), 355–359.

Smith, Russell E. "The Principle of Cooperation in Catholic Thought." In Peter J. Cataldo and Albert S. Moraczewski, eds. *The Fetal Tissue Issue: Medical and Ethical Aspects* (Braintree, MA: Pope John Center, 1994), pp. 81–92.

Smitz, J. et al. "Incidence of Severe Ovarian Hyperstimulation Syndrome after GnRH Agonist/HMG Superovulation for In-Vitro Fertilization." *Human Reproduction* 5 (1990), 933–937.

Soltor, Davor, and John Gearhart. "Enhanced: Putting Stem Cells to Work." *Science* 282/5407 (1999), 1468–1470.

Spinnato, Joseph A. "Mechanism of Action of Intrauterine Contraceptive Devices and Its Relation to Informed Consent." *American Journal of Obstetrics and Gynecology* 176/3 (1997), 503–506.

Stansberry, J. "The Infertile Couple: An Overview of Pathophysiology and Diagnostic Evaluation for the Primary Care Clinician." *Nurse Practitioner Forum* 7/2 (1996), 76–86.

Steghaus-Kovac, Sabine. "Biomedical Research: Ethical Loophole Closing Up for Stem Cell Researchers." *Science* 286 (1 October 1999), 31.

Steinbock, Bonnie. *Life Before Birth: The Moral and Legal Status of Embryos and Fetuses* (Oxford: Oxford University Press, 1992).

Steinbock, Bonnie. "Ethical Issues in Human Embryo Research." In National Institutes of Health, *Papers Commissioned for the Human Embryo Research Panel,* NIH Publication Number 95-3916 (Bethesda, MD: National Institutes of Health, 1994a), vol. 2, pp. 27–50.

Steinbock, Bonnie, and R. McClamrock. "When is Birth Unfair to the Child?" *Hastings Center Report,* 24/6 (1994b), 15–21.

Steinbock, Bonnie. "Respect for Human Embryos." In Paul Lauritzen, ed. *Cloning and the Future of Embryo Research* (New York: Oxford University Press, 2001), pp. 21–33.

Stillman, R. J. "In Utero Exposure to Diethylstilbestrol: Adverse Effects on the Reproductive Tract and Reproductive Performance in Male and Female Offspring." *American Journal of Obstetrics and Gynecology* 142 (1982), 905–921.

Stone, Jim. "Why Potentiality Matters." *Canadian Journal of Philosophy* 17/4 (1987), 815–830.

Stolberg, Sheryl Gay. "Stem Cell Research Advocates in Limbo," *The New York Times,* 20 January 2001, online edition: http://www.nytimes.com/2001/01/20/health/20stem/html.

Strain, Lisa, John C. S. Dean, Mark P. R. Hamilton, and David T. Bonthron. "A True Hermaphrodite Chimera Resulting from Embryo Amalgamation after In Vitro Fertilization." *New England Journal of Medicine* 338/3 (1998), 166–169.

Szebik, Imre. "Response to 'Germ Line Therapy to Cure Mitochondrial Disease: Protocol and Ethics of In Vitro Ovum Nuclear Transplantation by Donald. S. Rubenstein, David C. Thomasma, Eric A. Schon, and Michael J. Zinaman,'" *Cambridge Quarterly of Healthcare Ethics* 8 (1999), 369–374.

Tauer, Carol A. "Preimplantation Embryos, Research Ethics, and Public Policy." *Bioethics Forum,* 11/3, 1995, p. 30–37.

Tauer, Carol A. "Bringing Embryos into Existence for Research Purposes." In Nick Fotion and Jan C. Heller, eds., *Contingent Future Persons* (Dordrecht: Kluwer Academic Publishers, 1997), pp. 171–189.

Tauer, Carol A. "Private Ethics Boards and Public Debate." *Hastings Center Report* 29/2 (March–April 1999), 43–45.

Taunton-Rigby, Alison. "Testimony of Alison Taunton-Rigby, Ph.D., President and CEO, Aquila Biopharmaceuticals, Worcester, Massachusetts, on Behalf of the Biotechnology Industry Organization (BIO) Before the Subcommittee on Technology, Committee on Science. U.S. House of Representatives, Legislative Proposals Regarding Cloning Human Beings, July 22, 1997."

Thompson, Judith J. "A Defense of Abortion." *Philosophy and Public Affairs* 1/1 (1971), 47–77.

Thomson, James A. et al. "Embryonic Stem Cell Lines Derived from Human Blastocysts." *Science* 282 (6 November 1998), 1145–1147.

Tooley, Michael. "Abortion and Infanticide." *Philosophy and Public Affairs* 2/1 (Fall 1972), 37–65.

Travis, John. "Great Eggspectations: A Woman Is Born with 7 Million Protoeggs, of which Only 400 or So Will Mature and Be Capable of Being Fertilized. Now Researchers Are Trying to Create a Vast Supply of Human Eggs." *The Gazette* (Montreal), 24 May 1997, p. 18.

U.S. Congress, Office of Technology Assessment. *Infertility: Medical and Social*

Choices. OTA-BA-358 (Washington, DC: U.S. Government Printing Office, May 1988).

Underwood, Meredith, Elizabeth G. Harrison, William R. LaFleur, and Ronald M. Green. "Articles, Review Essay, and Response on the Theme 'Abortion and *Mizuko Kuyō* in Japan.'" *Journal of the American Academy of Religion* 67/4 (1999), 727–823.

Vaheri, A. et al. "Isolation of Attenuated Rubella-Vaccine Virus from Human Products of Conception and Uterine Cervix." *New England Journal of Medicine* 286/20 (1972), 1071–1074.

Van Steirteghem, André C. "Outcomes of Assisted Reproductive Technology." *New England Journal of Medicine* 383 (1998), 194–195.

Vatican, Congregation for the Doctrine of the Faith. "Donum Vitae: Instruction on Respect for Human Life in Its Origin and on the Dignity of Procreation." *Origins* 16/40 (17 March 1987), 697–711.

Veatch, Robert M. *The Basics of Bioethics* (Upper Saddle River, NJ: Prentice Hall, 1999).

Vogel, Gretchen. "Breakthrough of the Year: Capturing the Promise of Youth." *Science* 286 (17 December 1999), 2238–2239.

Vogel, Gretchen. "Company Gets Rights to Cloned Human Embryos." *Science* 287 (28 January 2000), 559.

Wade, Nicholas. "Researchers Claim Embryonic Cell Mix of Human and Cow." *New York Times,* 12 November, 1998, p. A1.

Wade, Nicholas. "Advisory Panel Votes for Use of Embryonic Cells in Research." *New York Times,* 29 June, 1999, p. A13.

Warnock, Mary. *A Question of Life: The Warnock Report on Fertilisation and Embryology* (Oxford: Basil Blackwell, 1985).

Warren, Mary Anne. "On the Moral and Legal Status of Abortion," *The Monist* 57/1 (January 1973), 43–61.

Warren, Mary Anne. "Do Potential People Have Moral Rights?" *Canadian Journal of Philosophy,* 7 (1977), 275–289.

Warren, Mary Anne. *Moral Status: Obligations to Persons and Other Living Things* (New York: Oxford University Press, 1997).

Washington, Harriet. "Vital Signs: Infertility Crisis Defies Stereotypes," *Emerge,* June 1998, p. 30.

Watt, Helen. "Potential and the Early Human." *Journal of Medical Ethics* 22 (1996), 222–226.

White, Gladys B. "Foresight, Insight, Oversight." *Hastings Center Report* 29/2 (March–April 1999), 41–42.

Wilcox, L. S., J. L. Kiely, C. L. Melvin, and M. C. Martin. "Assisted Reproductive Technologies: Estimates of Their Contribution to Multiple Births and Newborn Hospital Days in the United States." *Fertility and Sterility* 65 (1996), 361–366.

Wilkins-Haug, L. E., M. S. Rein, and M. D. Hornstein. "Oligospermic Men: The Role of Karyotype Analysis Prior to Intracytoplasmic Sperm Injection." *Fertility and Sterility* 67 (1997), 612–614.

Willadsen, S. M. "The Developmental Capacity of Blastomeres from 4- and 8-Cell Sheep Embryos." *Journal of Embryology and Experimental Morphology* 65 (1981), 165–172.

Willadsen, S. M. "Cloning of Sheep and Cow Embryos." *Genome* 31 (1989), 956–962.

Williams, Bernard. "Which Slopes Are Slippery?" In Michael P. Lockwood, ed., *Moral*

Dilemmas in Modern Medicine (Oxford: Oxford University Press, 1985), pp. 126–137.

Wilmut, I. "Cloning for Medicine." *Scientific American,* 279/6 (December 1998), 58–63.

Wilmut I. et al. "Viable Offspring Derived from Fetal and Adult Mammalian Cells." *Nature* 385 (1997), 810–813.

Wilmut, Ian, Keith Campbell, and Colin Tudge. *The Second Day of Creation* (New York: Farrar, Straus and Giroux, 2000).

Woodward, J. "The Non-Identity Problem." *Ethics* 96 (1986), 804–831.

Wymelenberg, S., for the Institute of Medicine (1990). *Science and Babies* (Washington, DC: National Academy Press, 1990).

Youngner, S. J., R. M. Arnold, and R. Schapiro. *The Definition of Death: Contemporary Controversies* (Baltimore: Johns Hopkins University Press, 1999).

Zaner, Richard M., ed. *Death: Beyond Whole-Brain Criteria* (Dordrecht: Kluwer Academic Publishers, 1988).

Zitner, Aaron. "Embryo Stem Cell Work Could Get Public Funding." *Los Angeles Times,* 13 August 2000, p. A1.

Appendix A
Stages of Embryonic Development*

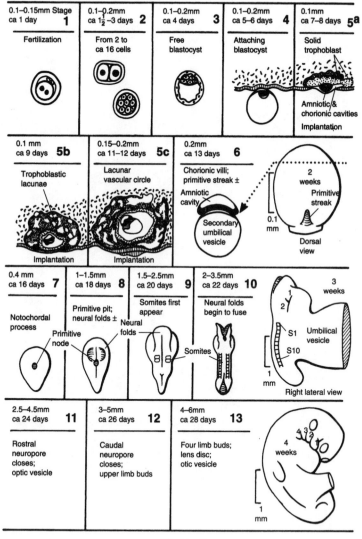

Figure A

*From Ronan O'Rahilly and Fabiola Müller, *Human Embryology & Teratology* (New York: Wiley-Liss, 1992). Reprinted by permission.

Appendix B
National Institutes of Health Human Embryo Research Panel: Categories of Research

Acceptable for Federal Funding

A research proposal is presumed acceptable if it is in accordance with the guidelines described earlier and is not described below as warranting additional review or being unacceptable. A protocol not in the last two categories would be classified acceptable if it is scientifically valid and meritorious; relies on prior adequate animal studies and, where appropriate, studies on human embryos without transfer; uses a minimal number of embryos; documents that informed consent will be obtained from acceptable donor sources; involves no purchase or sale of gametes or embryos; does not continue beyond the time of the usual appearance of the primitive streak in vivo (14 days); and has passed the required review by a local IRB, appropriate NIH study section and council, and, for the immediate future, the additional review body at the national level established at the discretion of the NIH Director.

Proposals in the acceptable category must also meet the specific guidelines set forth in this report concerning types of research (i.e., transfer, no transfer, parthenogenesis) (see chapter 5), and acceptable sources of gametes and embryos. Examples of such proposals include, but are not limited to:

- Studies aimed at improving the likelihood of a successful outcome for a pregnancy.
- Research on the process of fertilization.
- Studies on egg activation and the relative role of paternally-derived and maternally-derived genetic material in embryo development (parthenogenesis without transfer).
- Studies in oocyte maturation or freezing followed by fertilization to determine developmental and chromosomal normality.
- Research involving preimplantation genetic diagnosis, with and without transfer.

- Research involving the development of embryonic stem cells but only with embryos resulting from IVF for infertility treatment or clinical research that have been donated with the consent of the progenitors.
- Nuclear transplantation into an enucleated, fertilized or unfertilized (but activated) egg, without transfer, for research that aims to circumvent or correct an inherited cytoplasmic defect.

With regard to the last example, a narrow majority of the Panel believed such research should be acceptable for Federal funding. Nearly as many thought that the ethical implications of research involving the transplantation of a nucleus, whether transfer was contemplated or not, need further study before the research could be considered acceptable for Federal funding.

In addition to these examples, the Panel singled out two types of acceptable research for special consideration in the recommended ad hoc review process.

- Research involving the use of existing embryos where one of the progenitors was an anonymous gamete source who received monetary compensation. (This exception would apply only to embryos already in existence at the time at which this report is accepted by the Advisory Committee to the Director, NIH, should such acceptance occur.)
- A request to fertilize ova where this is necessary for the validity of a study that is potentially of outstanding scientific and therapeutic value.

In the first instance, for reasons explained in chapter 4 of this report, the Panel, with the exception of one member (see Appendix C) would make an allowance for an interim period for research involving the use of existing embryos where one of the progenitors was anonymous and had received monetary compensation. However, the Panel believes that in order to determine whether the exception might apply, special attention must be given during the review process to ensure that payment has not been provided for the embryo itself and that all other proposed guidelines are met.

In the second instance, Panel members believe that special attention is warranted for such research because of concern that attempts might be made to create embryos for reasons that relate solely to the scarcity of embryos remaining from infertility programs and because of the Panel's interest in preventing the creation of embryos for any but the most compelling reasons.

Warrants Additional Review

The Panel places research of a particularly sensitive nature in this category. The Panel did not make a determination for the acceptability of these proposals, and therefore recommends that there be a presumption against Federal funding of such research for the foreseeable future. This presumption could be overcome only by an extraordinary showing of scientific or therapeutic merit, together with explicit consideration of the ethical issues and social consequences. Such research proposals could be funded only after review by a broad-based ad hoc body created at the discretion of the Director, NIH, or by some other formal review process.

Research that the Panel determined should be placed in a category warranting additional review includes the following:

- Research between the appearance of the primitive streak and the beginning of neural tube closure.
- Cloning by blastomere separation or blastocyst splitting without transfer.
- Nuclear transplantation into an enucleated, fertilized or unfertilized (but activated) egg, with transfer, with the aim of circumventing or correcting an inherited cytoplasmic defect.
- Research involving the development of embryonic stem cells from embryos fertilized expressly for this purpose. (One member of the Panel dissents from this categorization; see appendix B.)
- Research that uses fetal oocytes for fertilization without transfer.

The Panel wishes to note that it was extremely circumspect in its consideration of the appropriate classification of the last two research areas and that members were divided in their views about where to place the research. For research involving the development of embryonic stem cells from deliberately fertilized oocytes, a narrow majority of members agreed such research warranted further review. A number of other members, however, felt that the research was acceptable for Federal funding, while some believed that such research should be considered unacceptable for Federal funding. The Panel's deliberation about the use of fetal oocytes for research without transfer involved painstaking reflection about the ethical implications and public sensibilities. The decision to recommend that this research be placed in the further review category, rather than the unacceptable category, was made by a bare majority.

Unacceptable For Federal Funding

Four ethical considerations entered into the deliberations of the Panel as it determined what types of research were unacceptable for Federal funding: the potential adverse consequences of the research for children, women and men; the respect due the preimplantation embryo; concern for public sensitivities about highly controversial research proposals; and concern for the meaning of humanness, parenthood, and the succession of generations.

Throughout its report the Panel considered these concerns as well as the scientific promise and the clinical and therapeutic value of proposed research, particularly as it might contribute to the well-being of women, children, and men. Regarding the types of research considered unacceptable, the Panel determined that the scientific and therapeutic value was low or questionable, or that animal studies did not warrant progressing to human research.

Research proposals in the unacceptable category should not be funded for the foreseeable future. Even if claims were made for their scientific or therapeutic value, serious ethical concerns counsel against supporting such research. Such research includes the following:

- Cloning of human preimplantation embryos by separating blastomeres or dividing blastocysts (induced twinning), followed by transfer in utero.
- Studies designed to transplant embryonic or adult nuclei into an enucleated egg, including nuclear cloning, in order to duplicate a genome or to increase the number of embryos with the same genotype with transfer.
- Research beyond the onset of closure of the neural tube.
- Research involving the fertilization of fetal oocytes with transfer.
- Preimplantation genetic diagnosis for sex selection, except for sex-linked genetic diseases.
- Development of human-nonhuman and human-human chimeras with or without transfer.
- Cross-species fertilization, except for clinical tests of the ability of sperm to penetrate eggs.
- Attempted transfer of parthenogenetically activated human eggs.
- Attempted transfer of human embryos into nonhuman animals for gestation.
- Transfer of human embryos for extrauterine or abdominal pregnancy.

INDEX

Abortion, 147, 187*n*. 165, 196*n*. 321
  and the beginning of human life,
    xii, 7
  and moral status of the embryo, 22–24,
    48–49
  opposition to, xii–xiii, 3, 57, 59, 77, 90,
    103, 106, 146–148, 153, 158–159,
    167, 171, 173–174, 199*n*. 371. *See
    also* Embryo research, opposition to
    by anti-abortion activists; Pro-life
    constituency
  right to, 21, 67. *See also* Pro-choice con-
    stituency; Reproductive liberty
  use of, for genetic reasons, 8, 57–59
  as women's only choice, in face of inade-
    quate contraceptives, 75
Acrosome reaction, 27
Activated egg. *See* Egg activation
Advanced Cell Technology, 137, 161, 177–
  78, 195*n*. 308
American Academy for the Advancement of
  Science (AAAS) working group, 86,
    138–39, 141, 146, 154, 156–57,
    173
  composition of, 139. *See also individual
    members' names*
Amniocentesis, 57
Andrews, Lori, 21, 31
Animal models, limits of, 119
Animal research, 8, 10, 55–56, 74, 98, 100,
    118–20, 148, 156, 171, 219, 222. *See
    also* Dolly (cloned sheep)
Animals, moral status of, 23–24, 50–51,
    172
Annas George, 79–80
Aronson, Diane, 4, 12
Artificial-natural distinction, 143–44
Assisted hatching, 9–11

Assisted reproductive technologies (ARTs),
    79. *See also* Infertility; Infertility
    medicine; *In vitro* fertilization
  opposition to, 11–12
Attractive egg, 183*n*. 87
Australian legislation, 3, 40, 86
Autologous, stem cell lines, definition of, 80

Balancing judgments, role of, in status de-
    terminations, 39, 143, 157. *See also*
    Decision, role of, in identification of
    biological markers; Reflective
    equilibrium
Ban on embryo research. *See* Embryo re-
    search, ban on
Ban on payment for gametes or embryos
    donated for research, 82–83
Biological individuation, 28–32, 36, 92
Birth control. *See* Contraception
Birth defects, x, xi, 8, 10, 16, 40–41, 69, 74,
    75, 77, 83, 96, 121, 125, 127–30
  epidemic of, as consequence of absence
    of embryo research, xii
Blastocyst, 7, 134, 136–37, 217. *See also*
    Embryo
  division of, 97, 100. *See also* Induced
    twinning
Blastomere, 7, 23, 28–31, 58
Blastomere separation, 29, 97, 99, 190*n*.
    217, 221–22. *See also* Cloning
Bonnicksen, Andrea, 115, 139
Boundary markers. *See also* Balancing judg-
    ments, role of, in status determina-
    tions choice-based nature of;
    Decision, role of, in identification of
    biological markers
  clarity and identifiability as criteria for
    choosing, 39–42, 63

223